Overcoming the Chronic Pain of Healthcare

I0115744

You never change things by fighting the existing reality.
To change something, build a new model that makes
the existing model obsolete.
– R. Buckminster Fuller

Overcoming the Chronic Pain of Healthcare

Keeping Safe in a System which can Kill, Harm, or Bankrupt You

Suzanne Fiscella, PA-C, MA, MS

ISBN: 978-1-7327566-0-1

Printed in the United States of America

Cover and interior design: Christy Collins, Constellation Book Services

This book is dedicated to my dad, Dr. Andre Fiscella, MD, and all his colleagues who spent years mentally digesting every part of the human body, learning every chemical reaction, every disease, every medication, and feeling the true joy in serving their patients. These men and women have given their lives to hours of study, spent thousands of dollars, taken out loans, and taken many a cold shower just to stay awake long enough to see another shift — these men and women who gave up their families for their careers, who found joy in being with their patients, who understood that every heart has a story and every story has meaning. These dedicated men and women continue to show up in the confines of windowless exam rooms, risking exposure to blood, sweat, and tears, heart, and soul to help a less fortunate human being. They cross borders of religion, color, politics, and race with no prejudice. They make no judgment about lifestyles and outcomes. Their only focus is on the human heart and how they can make it hope again when disease strikes. Their stethoscope is a listening tool for the story of a life held within the patient. Their patients' fears, anxiety, sadness, and survival are heard with every beat of the heart. They bring direction, comfort, and peace to those they serve.

My dad knew and loved his patients so very much. His inspiration and joy bring back memories of what true medicine is all about.

Note from the Author

Contents

PART 1

How We Got Here

CHAPTER 1

The Chronic Pain of Healthcare

If you are frustrated by the medical healthcare system we have today, you are not alone. Many folks have tried to navigate the system, purchasing large amounts of insurance at very high premiums, settling for large deductibles only to find that when payment comes due, they still owe exorbitant amounts over and above what they have already paid. Add to that the fact that, when you call for an appointment for something as urgent as a worrisome mole you just noticed, a headache that won't go away, or numbness in your feet or hands, your worry is escalated when the call center operator tells you the first available appointment will be three to four weeks away.

As healthcare consumers, we try to take care of ourselves; we try to eat healthfully and exercise when we can. We are busy with our marriages, our careers, raising our families, taking care of our aging parents, volunteering in the community to help others less fortunate than us. Then why are we settling for high insurance premiums and poor service? Why are we not getting the same customer care that we expect, the service we want?

When we go to a restaurant, purchase a cup of coffee, or go to a movie, do we return if the service or product was not what we expected? We're used to a drive-through where we can get something quickly, express lines for checking out, apps on our phone to get us a ride in three minutes, punching a button and having something delivered to our door within one day. Shouldn't healthcare be the same? Shouldn't you have access to healthcare when you need it? Certainly the fees and the prices that you pay in healthcare should afford you better service, better outcomes, and the care you expect.

We all believe that obtaining needed, quality healthcare should not be this hard. But then we also think our marriages, raising our children, taking care of our aging parents, and our careers shouldn't be this hard either. But they are. So, what do we do when life overwhelms us? To whom do we turn? How do we get through those moments? We somehow manage to get back on track. Our downs begin to disappear, and our ups begin to rise once again.

Our health is no different. It has its ups. It has its downs. When we suffer the loss of a loved one, the experience brings fear that perhaps we should get a check-up. When our children are sick, we worry. When our parents need care and can't afford it, we become frustrated. One of the things we expect in healthcare is good care. We expect the best. We expect choices and options. We want to know that our doctors are taking care of us. We want our doctors to partner with us. But the old ways of easy healthcare are difficult to find in today's healthcare model.

It is difficult to find ways to navigate a complicated system. We have to ask the right questions. Healthcare made easy? It seems the healthcare system is only complicating things more.

This book is going to guide you through the steps to simplify the healthcare process. After years of practicing medicine, turning to advocacy work, and having the experience of knowing what the pre-insurance era of medicine looked like, I have come up with a system that works and want to share it with you. What follows is a framework of how we got bad, incompetent healthcare today and how you can fix it, regardless of what you are struggling with. This will lay the foundation. It gives you a solid look at what healthcare was and why you are not the problem — the system is. The key is clarity — asking the right questions, going into healthcare with preparation and certainty.

How do patient advocates know this works? Because we have helped thousands of patients and their doctors get back to clarity, options, and conversation about what works and doesn't work and what's best for you.

The second part of this book will break down healthcare into six aspects. Each aspect has its own set of questions, concerns, and roadmaps for you to educate yourself with. Each aspect can be customized to fit your needs. This customization begins a powerful journey for you to obtain the treatment choices that are out there waiting for you. Whether you are handling healthcare for your children, your aging parents, or your friends, you can customize their healthcare plan to meet their needs, not the needs of the healthcare system.

Each of these six aspects has certain rules. We will explore these rules. You will learn which medical documents are important for you to carry to every doctor's office, which questions to ask, and how to know you are getting the right treatment options.

Most of us can get through life handling the minor problems that come our way. For example, the lightbulb goes out. We buy a new lightbulb and replace the old one. But when all the lights in the house start flickering and you smell wires burning, it's time to call in a professional. Likewise, this book will show you when your customized health plan needs a professional patient advocate to guide you through unanswered, confusing roadblocks and the costs of healthcare.

The third part of this book will guide you to the right professionals, including patient advocates, doctors, and surgeons. You will learn when to reach out for the advice and roadmap you need. After reading this book, you will no longer be held hostage by a system of smoke and mirrors. Clarity will come to you at every turn. You will be treated like the respected consumer you are.

Doctors are leaving the healthcare system in order to reconnect with their patients. These dedicated men and women and their evolving responses to the healthcare system will be discussed in chapter 14.

When the roadblocks are too great, it's time to call in the right certified patient advocate. Because this new, emerging profession is so fast-growing, terminology and definitions have not been clarified. For now, we will use general terms. A certified patient advocate is an independent business owner with his or her own practice in patient advocacy. They work strictly for the client or patient, who pays them directly for their services. They do not take insurance. You or your family will pay only for the service you need and not keep paying a monthly fee like insurance payments. Think of one as you would a real estate agent you may have used in the past. He or she helped you sell your home. They work for themselves in their own real estate practice. They help you navigate through murky transactions in real estate. Certified patient advocates help you navigate through the murky healthcare system.

While this book will teach you how to advocate for yourself, prevent medical error, and safely get back to your normal health, there may be times you need additional guidance. Certified patient advocates work to prevent healthcare errors as well as fix them after they occur. When you don't have the energy to clarify all that confuses you, your advocate becomes your guide. He or she picks up where you leave off and leads you to the healthcare services you deserve. The patient advocate steps in to discern exactly what your healthcare goals are, which services you need, and what your end result can look like. Getting you through worry and grief is hard enough. Add to this the fact that the roadmap used in healthcare is often incomplete, the wrong map, or just outdated. Patient advocates know how to find your right map, the right services, the options, the best care. They are well trained in the twists and turns you're going to encounter. They are also experts in putting up the guardrails, keeping you safe, telling you when to slow down and when to speed up, directing you against wrong turns and dead ends. To find Board-Certified Patient Advocates you can go to www.PatientBest.com.

Let's look at how frustrating healthcare service can be by using an analogy:

Imagine yourself getting ready for a lovely dinner date. You called ahead and reserved a table at a fine restaurant (your appointment). You get there on time and the hostess tells you it will still be an hour — the kitchen (doctor) is running late. Then you wait for a menu but you never get one. When you inquire about it, your waitress tells you do not need one. The kitchen (doctor) knows what's best for you. You ask about prices and are told nobody knows them. Your server (nurse) finally asks you what you feel like eating (why you are there to see your doctor) and you still wait another hour for your food — the kitchen (doctor) is still running late. So you are not told the prices, and when you try to get help, your server tells you to talk to the kitchen (your doctor, who has no idea what you are there for). If the food (medicine) you are given is not to your liking, your restaurant tells you there are no refunds (prescriptions cannot be taken back). Would you seriously go back to a service like this again?

This is a perfect example of healthcare today. Your appointment time should be your reserved time to meet with the doctor, not a time to begin waiting another hour or two. No one knows your body better than you do, but all the choices you could utilize if you knew they existed are never discussed. The unknown prices are what you may or may not pay depending on what your insurance deems appropriate. Later, when you call someone for help with your high, unexplained bills, you are told to call another department. Yet Americans flock to their doctor's office over and over again, only to be met with resistance caused by time constraints, production quotas, and patient satisfaction surveys, all of which a broken healthcare system demands of their doctors.

Let's get you the services you need when you need them. Let's make healthcare transparent and expect better service at a price you can afford. Since we have to live (or die) at the hands of our healthcare system, learn how to stay away from common mistakes and where to get better choices, and then hire a professional when the situation so demands.

There are a few fundamentals we need to establish first and concepts to master before we start. We'll cover these in chapter 2.

CHAPTER 2

The "Medicine versus Healthcare" Conflict

Most folks confuse "medicine" with "healthcare," often thinking they are synonymous. They are two separate entities. Years ago, there was *only* medicine. It is critical that you understand what medicine used to look like in the old days to comprehend the gargantuan difference between that and today's healthcare system. It is also important to understand that "healthcare" is short for "healthcare business." Somewhere along the quiet trail of economic growth and prosperity, healthcare business weaved itself into every doctor-patient relationship, leaving both doctor and patient wondering what happened. Let's look at what medicine looked like before healthcare business and what it looks like today. Only then can you understand the difference.

First, know that medicine is better than it has ever been. There are better procedures, cures, medications, research, and understanding than ever before. We are curing cancer in many parts of the medical world, HIV medications are more advanced than ever, and the da Vinci Robot has brought technology to its ultimate expression in surgery.[1] The good news is that you don't have to learn medicine in this book. Your doctors, physician assistants, and nurse practitioners went to school to learn medicine and its terminology for you. They are required to keep up with the latest and best approaches in medicine. They have committed their time and vast amounts of money dedicating themselves to your world of medicine. They have learned the language and speak it to one another. Again, this is good news. They practice with passion and they love working with you, the patient.

But wait a minute. You know frustrations, confusion, fear, and anger. Again, medicine and healthcare are two different entities. The frustration, confusion, fear, and anger you feel are a result of the healthcare business system. With so many new players and moving parts, our healthcare business system is convoluted and fragmented and has destroyed the doctor-patient relationship.

When I work in the urgent care clinic, patients will complain to me, "I called my doctor's office and couldn't get in today, so I had to come here. They said it would be three weeks before I could see my doctor." Okay. Time for new language. You did not call "your doctor's office"; you called "your healthcare business office." There is no such thing as a "doctor's office" anymore unless your physician runs a practice by her- or himself and is not part of a healthcare business. Doctors are just as frustrated. They, like you, discourage their children from going into the medical field these days.

So let's look at what medicine was and how healthcare business has roadblocked your relationship with your doctor. As an illustration, my personal story with medicine versus healthcare business will empower you to win the war on healthcare, too.

It was December and I was only eleven years old. My life would change. My dad was a family practice doctor and his office was in the front part of our home. We lived in a small community in upstate New York.

This day began no differently than any other. I was getting ready for school. My mom and five siblings were busy getting ready as well and running around the house looking for books and lunches. Dad's office hours began at seven a.m. and ended at eight p.m. every weekday. He took Wednesday afternoon off but worked Saturday mornings. He was on call twenty-four/seven. On this cold, gray morning, he came in through our back door after making his rounds at the hospital. He saw me sitting at the kitchen table and sat down next to me. His next words would signal the first of two events that led me to help so many frustrated patients find help in health services today.

He said, "How would you like to work in my office?" I jumped at the chance. It wasn't so much that I loved medicine but that I just loved being around my dad. He loved to laugh and tell jokes. His family and his patients loved him for his excellent care, nonjudgmental way, and easy laugh.

So, why did Dad pick me out of his six children? When I was four, Dad would come out of his office, stand in our kitchen, and announce he had to go see a patient. Another house call. Who wanted to go with him? He would look at all us kids, and I would be the first to jump at the chance to go with my dad. He didn't seem to mind. So off I went doing house calls with the man in a tie and jacket, holding the big black bag.

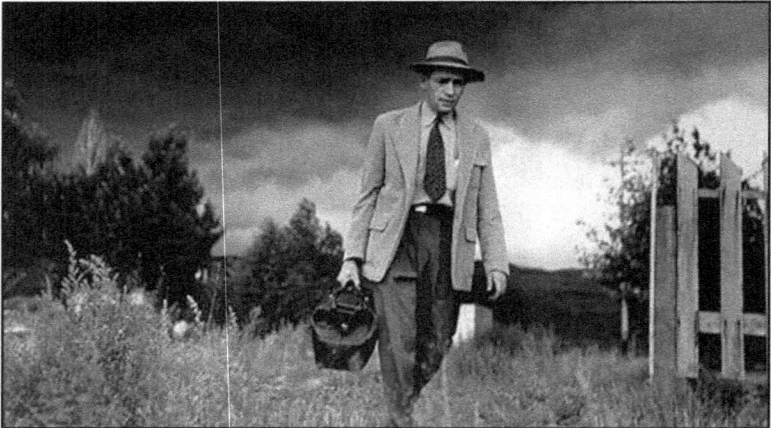

Dr. Earnest Ciani, Colorado, 1942; a typical image of a physician practicing medicine as we knew it up to the 1980s

I was afraid to go into these strange houses, but Dad reassured me, and I would sit in the living room on the plastic-covered couch and wait for him while he went into the bedroom. He would come out ten minutes later and whisper something to the spouse, who always seemed to lower his or her head in sadness, and then we would leave. Sometimes they would offer "Doc" food and he seemed to always eat. When we got in the car he would say, "Don't tell your Mother I just ate." And then he would eat again at the family dinner when we got home.

So, at eleven years old, I entered medicine. I worked with Dad most evenings through high school and then on and off when I returned home from college. I called patients in from the waiting room and led them to the chair by my dad's desk. Dad would take their blood pressure, listen to their hearts (with and without a stethoscope), and talk with them. During these office visits, doctor and patient each smoked a cigarette. Then the patient would get up and be led by me to another room, where they would pay the $4.00 office fee and leave through another door to our front porch. No one had insurance; we didn't even know what that was. Every once in a while, Dad would go behind the portable frame with a curtain and give the patient a shot. That was an extra dollar.

Dad's "medicine" didn't consist of just office visits or house calls. Every weekend, he would come out to our kitchen all dressed up in his nice blue suit and gather my mom, and off they would go to a patient's wedding, funeral, graduation, bar-mitzvah, bat-mitzvah, christening, or confirmation. He was never without events to go to on weekends.

Once I asked Dad why we had no charts, just a clipboard with patients' names on them for each day. He said, "Why do I need a chart? I know all my patients, their families; I know their hospitalizations because I see them when I round in the hospital early mornings. I know their drinking, smoking, and eating habits because I attend family celebrations and gatherings." Mom decided it was time to get charts, so we developed one sheet of paper with a name and date of birth on it. That was it. My job was to write down what Dad was ordering for them.

When Dad needed to order a medicine, he gave out paper prescriptions or called the pharmacist for some strange concoction. The pharmacist had a special telephone line in the back of the pharmacy for all the doctors, so my dad never had to wait on hold.

When Dad suspected a broken arm, he called the orthopedic doctor. The office would answer and immediately Dad would be connected to the doc. In fact, the orthopedic doctor was always called from a patient's exam room to speak with my dad. All Dad would say was, "Hey, Martin, it's Andre. I'm sending over a patient. I think he has a broken arm." Yep, that was it! Off the patient went. Dad never charged for these visits. The orthopedic doctor always seemed to call my dad back to let him know about his patient, what treatment his patient had received, and how his patient was recovering. Likewise, when a physician called, Dad stopped what he was doing and immediately took the call.

Medicine consisted of my dad's nurse during the normal day hours, a pharmacist he could call at any time, and a hospital he could visit any time. Yep, life was simple. If there was paperwork instead of conversation, I didn't see it.

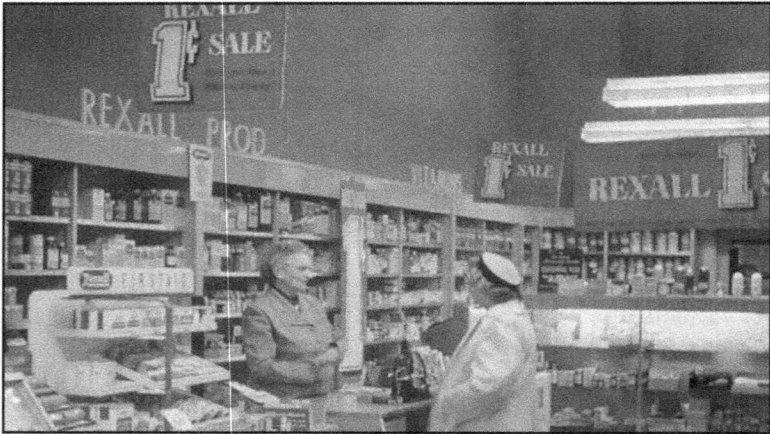

Typical pharmacy in the 1960s and '70s

Dad seemed to know so much about the patients and they loved him for it. He always knew about their families, their jobs, and who was going off to school or who was getting married. Medicine was more than just health issues. Medicine was counseling, listening, and giving the care we all expected. The doctor partnered with his patients. He or she was there to make life easier, more secure, and less frightening when those ups were disappearing and the downs were rearing their unwanted heads.

So now you know what medicine was like back in the '60s and '70s, with its simplicity and the special relationships doctors had with their patients. This glimpse into the past will hopefully give you a perspective from which to view the stark differences we have today.

It interesting to note that, in an age of quick, easily downloadable instant movies, drive-through fast-food restaurants, rides that can pick you up in less than five minutes, we have healthcare failing to follow suit. While other services in our lives have simplified, medicine has gone in the opposite direction.

Now, for the second reason I am writing this book. Dad assumed I would always go into medicine, but I thought he worked too hard and decided against it. I found out later that it wasn't "work" to him, but passion. My brother and sister, on the other hand, decided to go to medical school, and each has held a solo family practice since 1979. They have never sold out to healthcare business. They love working on their own like my Dad did.

I decided to become a teacher. One day, I was challenging my high school students. "What will you do after high school? What is your love, your passion? What fills your heart with joy? What is the one thing you could do and can't wait to do every day of your life?" I heard a small voice in the back of the room say, "What would you do if you hadn't become a teacher?" The words stuck, and I thought timidly, "I would become a physician assistant." I was fifty years old and not about to start medical school and residency. But I knew a physician assistant could see patients, write prescriptions, and work in medicine and that it was a 30-month program. Off to physician assistant (PA) school I went at age fifty.

When I graduated and started to practice, I knew something was drastically wrong. I had left medicine in 1979 and I never kept up with it after that. So, imagine my surprise when I saw all the changes in 2006! In 1979, medicine was easy and simple. My dad's practice, as well as all the other practices in town consisted of a pharmacist, a hospital, a nurse, and a family who took care of one another. Doctors called one another about their patients. Specialists knew which doctor referred which patient to them.

While medicine had advanced tremendously and new procedures, new medications, and new specialties abounded, what also had come with these changes was a heavy, smothering pressure called "healthcare business." It is made up of rules and regulations and big businesses whose purpose it is to "streamline medicine." While doctors were busy taking care of patients, this giant crept into their profession under the guise of "healthcare" and has overwhelmed patients and doctors since. Business policy and profit guidelines run your "doctor's office" today.

Healthcare business began as a totally new way of organizing but *not* practicing medicine. The one-on-one personal relationship was replaced with administration and government policy. When I saw how foreign medicine had become, I called my brother and sister to ask them what had happened to the profession. Two thoughts struck me. First, they had never worked in Dad's office, so they didn't see the personal relationship and time my dad gave his patients. Old medicine was about a special conversation between patient and doctor. Jerome Goodman, MD, says it best in his book *How Doctors Think* when he writes, "Language is still the bedrock of pinnacle practice."[2]

While my brother and sister know their patients and their families, they also now deal with a heavy healthcare system of mandates and requirements reaching deep into their private practices. They had grown up with the new managed-care medicine as we know it today, so they didn't notice the subtle changes and differences between managed care and the medicine my father had practiced. It was like putting a frog in cold water and turning up the heat slowly. Over time the frog will not notice and be cooked to death. I was like the frog who jumped into the pot of boiling water and scrambled to get out. I was seeing major complications, miscommunications, strangers working on patients, and worse, patients lost to a sea of frustration.

Leaving medicine twenty-seven years prior had left me with the feeling that personal conversation between patient and doctor was the number one reason anyone practiced medicine or served in the medical field. Now all I could see were six-minute appointments, strangers sitting on exam tables, and no communication between hospitals, doctors, specialists, labs, radiology centers, and patients and their families. Charts were supposed to be the one item that connected patients to their unfamiliar doctors, but they were either incomplete or wrong. Patients were frustrated with long wait times, insurance denials, and high premiums while at high risk to suffer a medical error because they did not know the system nor did their doctors personally know their patients. Talk about "stranger danger" in life — what about in the exam room?

Here is a glimpse of what healthcare business looks like today. Is it no wonder that patients are confused, scared, and frustrated when they can't get answers, on-time office visits, or medical treatment?

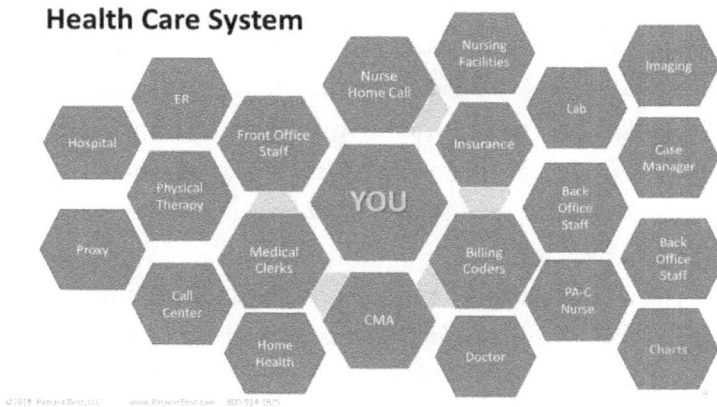

Health Care System

The list of new professions in medicine is overwhelming. Everyone and every company decided they needed to have a piece of the medical pie. No one really knew where to begin. No one was really talking to patients and finding out what their needs were. If the medical profession couldn't figure out a starting point and ending point in this myriad of healthcare, how could the patient?

When the National Patient Safety Foundation came out in 2013 with a study that medical error was the third leading cause of death in America today, behind heart disease and cancer, did patients take notice?[3] Johns-Hopkins noted similar studies.[4] With so many people running healthcare, who is in charge? You? The government? Your insurance company? Your doctor? It should be you. It's your health. It's your body and no two people react the same way to stress, life, and medical treatment. Healthcare big business cannot claim "one size fits all." We all react differently to our medical care. This is evident by the number of people who die at the hands of healthcare today.

Out of my three-week career in medicine came frustration and fear for my patients. Something had to be done. If I could teach the Pythagorean theorem to ninth-graders, I could certainly teach patients how to maneuver through the fragmented healthcare system of today. I could teach patients how to become informed participants in their own care. Did no one think about the dangers of our modern healthcare system? Patients didn't need to learn "medicine." Their doctors knew that. But I could teach patients how to master the rules to succeed in our healthcare system as we know it to be structured today. I could show them the landmines and give them the tools to partner with their compassionate and caring doctors, who have never wavered from the same commitment my dad showed his patients.

So my years of teaching kicked in and I began attacking the healthcare debacle through education. Patients were going to learn the tricks of the trade and the rules of the road. Off to the drawing board I went! There were plenty of books on healthy eating and exercise habits. We don't need to focus on that. This book is about how to demystify the system. How to get back to that doctor-patient relationship.

Think about it this way. When learning to drive, we just don't jump behind a wheel and start driving. We learn the rules of the road, what the signs mean, and what happens when we ignore those signs. We learn to be proactive and alert while driving. After months of practice, we are finally given a road test and then we are "competent" and ready to drive.

There are three new medical models entering the healthcare market. They are taking this country by storm. Patients and doctors are reaching across the healthcare abyss to rebuild the bridge of care and conversation that was once there. Both parties are seeing eye-to-eye again, clarifying treatment goals, and building friendships and trust in the exam room. Americans are realizing that if they are going to get the medical care and services they need and pay for, they will need to take control of their own destinies.

Model 1 is addressed in part 2 of this book. It is about owning your own set of medical records, cleaning up the mistakes you will find in them, getting in to see your physician in timely manner, and learning how to have a decent conversation with your doctor. Asking the right questions will give you a better outcome every time.

Model 2 augments Model 1. A new professional has emerged to help you and your loved ones when you feel overwhelmed, tired, or scared. The patient advocate has mastered and will help you navigate our chaotic healthcare system. From phone calls to set up appointments to medical bills that keep pouring in, these people know how to navigate around the snags. They clarify, find better treatment options, guide you and your aging parents, help you with your child's treatment, or keep you living at home longer and aging in place. At Patient Best® we have certified patient advocates, dedicated men and women who make a priority of safety, communication between their clients (you, the patient) and your doctors, and keeping options open at all times. They know the "tricks of the trade." They know the best doctors in town and, unfortunately, they know the worst ones, too. They find you the healthcare you deserve.

Model 3 is the direct primary care physician. While Americans are learning to overcome a poorly run healthcare system and patient advocates are emerging to help, doctors are also reaching across the healthcare abyss. More physicians are leaving big-business healthcare. In this model, patients pay for medical services directly. No insurance is needed. Costs are significantly less. In part 3 of this book, you will learn more about

Model 3 and the simplicity of it all. It's medicine made easy for those of us who are tired of confusion. It is written for those who want the secrets to healthy healthcare.

Staying out of the healthcare business system but finding the right primary care doctor to partner with is critical. When patients complain of bad knee replacements, painful back fusions, chronic pains, or twenty medicines, we see a system failing the patients. What makes some patients live to 104 happily and healthily while others crash and burn in their 80s? After years of working with a practice in which the average age of patients is 86, I have a few insights.

Now that we've defined the difference between medicine and healthcare, you can master your own healthcare. You will own it, work it, and be a significant player in obtaining the care you need when you need it. The services of your doctor and your own dedicated healthcare team are going to be built by you. And if you or your loved one runs into a snag and needs help navigating, then you can seek out a patient advocate.

Before you can navigate the healthcare system and begin taking control, you want to learn the basic rules of the healthcare road. Physicians have been using the same rules in practicing medicine for years. Now it is time for you to learn those rules so that you and your doctor can coordinate your efforts.

Let's go back to the driving analogy. Are we ready for *every* situation and *every* crazy driver that comes our way? No, but we develop the skill to protect ourselves from such mishaps. This is how this book is written. This approach will help you develop the skills you need to handle any mistakes that come your way. It will build that trusting doctor-patient relationship for you.

In partnering with your doctor, you have someone to help you through this maze. If you cannot find a doctor you can trust, then find a patient advocate to help you find one.

With most things in life, we learn the "rules of the road." Whether it's a new cell phone, new computer, new job, or new course, there are certain rules that, when followed, will make sense to the operator, new employee, or new student. When we get in a bind or cannot figure out the system, we turn to professional help to get us untangled from the mess we are in. If it's our phone or computer, that's simple — we just call a child. If it's a roof or electrical problem, we try to fix it first and then call a contractor.

You need to know that doctors and nurses are not at fault. They are not the ones breaking the system. Somehow, somewhere, healthcare business saw the opportunity to capitalize on medicine. When that crack of financial opportunity opened, the doctors were too busy taking care of patients to see the covert takeover. So blaming doctors is like blaming your cell phone when you have no service. It's a network issue, not your cell phone.

Let's get back to the good news — that the doctor-patient relationship is still the same caring and concerned relationship it was in the twentieth century. The "rules of the exam room" that all doctors follow are the same. You are going to learn these rules and re-form collaboration. There are certain skills that you can develop to enhance outcomes. Just as we all learned how to drive and to balance a checkbook, we can learn to master "patient-ability" anywhere.

And the better news is that your doctor will love you for it. Your doctor will give you time, the real pearl you spend together talking through concerns, plans, and fears. Trust solidifies rapport, and rapport begets respect.

If the fast-paced healthcare system has blindsided you, then it's time to be proactive. Learn each part of modern healthcare and how to prevent medical error or death while securing the best outcomes in recovery. Your doctors will embrace you for being a student of your healthcare. And yes, you will capture the doctor-patient relationship that once lived. It just got buried under the heavy, suffocating smoke and mirrors called big-business healthcare. But caring medicine is still breathing a shallow breath, with a barely beating pulse. You can give it life again.

Let's wake it up . . .

CHAPTER 3

Healthcare Errors

As mentioned in the previous chapter, The National Safety Foundation stated in 2013 that medical mistakes are the number three killer of Americans today, behind heart disease and cancer, and Johns-Hopkins has confirmed this conclusion. Anyone who has worked in healthcare will agree. Mistakes abound. The hardest information to obtain is the true number of deaths caused by healthcare and the number of patients whose lives have been changed because of medical error. The reason these numbers are so hard to find is that no one is counting. It is estimated that 260 to 400 thousand Americans die each year as a result of healthcare mistakes. If this is accurate, then about seven hundred to one thousand patients die every day, seven days a week. This is equivalent to two jumbo jets crashing every day.

Let's compare these figures with the airline industry. If two jumbo jets went down every day, seven days a week, how many of us would fly? Yet, we will fly to the healthcare office without giving pause to consider the healthcare mistakes that may meet us head-on.

Unlike the healthcare business, the National Safety Transportation Board (NTSB) is intent on finding errors and correcting them. In the event of a plane crash, they analyze every piece of equipment and scrutinize the crash site and the plane's black box. They don't stop there. They look at all events that led up to the crash. They then contact all airlines, telling them what went wrong and exploring ways to improve training and procedures so that the problem will be resolved and never occur again. Airlines crashes, like healthcare crashes, are usually the result multiple smaller errors that accumulate until the big one occurs. The NSTB will figure out their causes and keep our skies safe. Not so in healthcare. When a patient dies of a medical error or complications from a procedure, the death certificate does not reflect this. The healthcare industry is not notified, no new training occurs, and the problem goes unaddressed.

My friend's dad had surgery to have a pacemaker put in his heart. Three weeks later, he was short of breath. The problem was that he had two liters of "fluid" around the heart. The doctor put a needle into the chest to remove the fluid, which was interfering with the heart's ability to expand and contract with each beat. The heart had been punctured (no one knew) by the pacemaker. When the fluid was discovered to be blood, it was concerning, as the heart muscle was leaking blood with every contraction. This meant the heart had a hole that would need to be repaired. Medical staff, thinking it plausible to remove the blood and then repair the hole, inserted a syringe and drained the blood from the heart. Unfortunately, it was not a hole in the heart muscle but a tear. Having no pressure holding them together, the heart muscles ripped open and the patient died immediately. The death certificate said, "Heart failure."

Where's the National Healthcare Safety Board? Oh wait, there isn't one. Could that physician have gotten extra training? You bet. But did that occur? No. Did other physicians learn from this surgeon's mistake? No. Did the patient *really* die of heart failure?

This is not new information to most of us. When we are diagnosed with a disease or disorder, we should always look for that one doctor or clinic that specializes in the disease. If it's a surgery we must undergo, we look for that one doctor who has done hundreds of those procedures and is recommended by our friends. We know there are going to be risks. Can we minimize them? In most cases, yes, but only if we pay attention, ask the right questions, and speak up and get help when we know something is wrong.

As physician assistants, our profession allows us to train and often work with dozens of different physicians. We see the ones who have excellent skills and knowledge. We see those who have "no bedside manner" but are extremely knowledgeable in their specialties. We work with those who spend hours worrying about their patients and their families. We also get to see those who could use more training. There is a saying in medicine: "What do you get when you seek a second opinion? A second opinion." The joke here is that you never get the same opinion but a *different* opinion. Different doctors do practice medicine differently. In one ER (emergency room) where I worked, the doctor preferred a certain pain medicine, but when the next physician arrived for his shift we had to change the IV (intravenous) pain medication according to his preference.

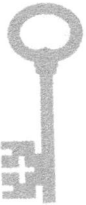

The key here is to find the provider you trust and have confidence in. Do your homework. We will talk more about how the system makes you, the consumer, feel like a fool when it comes to getting physician references. And we will guide you to the right doctors when you need them.

As a patient advocate, I have asked many patients why they are going back to the doctor. They have no clue. What is the expected outcome? Why does the doctor want to see you again? Most patients just rub their thumb and fingers together, indicating "Money." Even if patients do not ask why they are returning for a visit, certainly they ask why those responsible for procedures that have gone awry are not brought to justice.

No, they don't ask that either. Every once in a while a patient's family may get an attorney and sue the hospital, the doctor, and everyone who touched their loved one or was involved in the care of the patient. But at the end of the day, a gag order is placed on the family if they want to settle. The gag order is a "hush-hush" agreement that in effect says that it is okay for this to be done again and again to others. Do not blame the victims or their families. There is insurmountable pressure from defendants' attorneys bullying these victims into signing gag orders. Anyone who has ever brought charges or a lawsuit understands how they are threatened with "losing everything" if they insist on going to court. They are told, "You will never work in this field again. You will never work in this town again." "You will be ruined." Or, if the patient's family goes to court, they are told that they won't be seen by any doctors in the community. They are told no doctor will touch them because they publicly sued. So they sign the gag order to settle.

Look at all the men and women who have spoken up against sexual harassment, and yet the perpetrators can continue their abuse for years because of gag orders placed because of bullying by attorneys that left the victims in choke holds. In fact, one plaintiff's attorney said, "It is frowned upon to be in court instead of settling outside of court. If I keep bringing cases to an overworked judge, he or she gets mad at me and will not rule in my clients' favor. Then my reputation precedes me, and I don't get clients and I am out of work." So, to protect the wrongful actions of both provider and healthcare these "gag orders" are stamped into settlements to protect healthcare and medical mistakes. Let's face it, if an airline keeps crashing, well, you just can't hide that from the media. When a patient dies of a medical mistake, well, call it heart failure and let the incompetent system carry on.

Healthcare systems have been called on the carpet for not providing better care. But how can a business give better service when its focus is on the dollar? Recently, a new mandate was implemented that directed healthcare systems to do surveys of their patients. These patient satisfaction surveys meant the difference between payment or penalty. Naturally, the healthcare systems took notice. Doctors and front-line healthcare workers had better do a better job and satisfy their patients so patient satisfaction surveys will be positive.

> One doctor I spoke with had twelve excellent reviews and three bad reviews, so she had to meet with the patient-centered-care director. She said the director told her to improve her listening skills, spend more time with each patient, and give a pamphlet to each patient. The pamphlet told the patients that they would be getting a survey and to please tell the doctor before they leave the office whether they are dissatisfied with their care, so the doctor could address any problems ahead of time, before the survey was emailed, ensuring a good review for the clinic.
>
> The doctor then went on to say that she was still given ten-minute appointments with each patient; so how was she to fit any of this additional activity in?

Patients need to understand the depth of despair and frustration every front-line medical provider and doctor feels within his or her work environment. Hospital nurses are overworked. Caring for twenty very ill patients a day and then managing charts, chasing down hospitalists (physicians who treat you in the hospital), and answering to families can be exhausting. Hospitals are often short-staffed, with nurses and CMAs (certified medical assistants) covering for the shortage, receptionists answering phone calls and fielding angry patients, and insurance companies not authorizing doctor-ordered tests. We can't begin to list all the healthcare providers in the industry who work day and night without breaks to help a patient. These men and women have amazed me endlessly. I have seen machines break, instruments fall, patients faint, and yet, no matter what profession providers are in, they truly know how to respond to a situation or patient gone bad. These are the men and women who in times of disaster will run toward devastation and destruction to save a life, at the risk of losing their own. Yet, the administration running dollar-induced healthcare is rarely seen on the front lines, where the passion is. Is it no wonder the burnout in healthcare is at an all-time high?

So let's talk about your healthcare office visit and how patients can give healthcare personnel a patient they dream about. When we take responsibility for our healthcare acumen, our healthcare system will have to rise to our expectations, not preserve their own.

We will sit in a waiting room for hours to be seen for only ten minutes but will never ask the front desk what's taking so long. If traffic slows on the highway, you can bet we are on our cell phones looking up the GPS news to see what's taking so long with the traffic ahead of us. Do restaurants have waiting rooms? Where else is one told they have an appointment only to arrive on time and find out they will wait two hours. When airplanes announce a delay in flights, the moaning is heard miles away. Why do we not do this at the doctor's office? We have been conditioned to wait in doctors' offices when technology gives us speed and accuracy in every other profession. Would you wait hours to be served at a restaurant when you had called ahead and reserved a table? Probably not, so why do you wait hours to see your doctor when you have an appointment? Shouldn't waiting rooms be obsolete with today's fast-paced technology? They are, in direct primary care offices, which we will talk more about in part 3.

Here in this chapter, we will explore healthcare mistakes that are seen repeatedly. You will learn to recognize the signs and avoid them. There are fourteen main critical errors in healthcare business that must be avoided. These errors are not committed by one person. They are constellations of mistakes that make it through the system when most of us don't know the healthcare driving rules and how we can change them.

Healthcare Mistake 1. Medications

Medications account for 77 percent of all medical mistakes. Because medications come with a long list of rules, at any junction in the medication highway miscommunication can easily occur. Let's look at the questions to be addressed when taking medications:

→ When do I take it?

→ How long do I take it?

→ What is it for?

→ What are the side effects?

→ For what side effects should I call the office?

→ If I get a side effect, can I just stop the medication, or do I have to gradually reduce it?

→ Do I take it with or without food?

→ Will milk or juice block its absorption?

→ Can I take my vitamins with it?

→ Do I have to take it the same time every day?

→ Do I take it at the same time I take other medications?

→ How will I know if the medication is working?

→ When will I start to feel better?

We will dedicate a whole chapter to medications and will address possilbe mistakes. Suffice it to say that, because medications have so many aspects, using them safely without all the necessary information may be like try putting together a bicycle with a part missing. The result may be a disaster, just as the bike may become unsafe.

Mistake 2. Miscommunications

If you have ever been married, then you must know that what you say and what your spouse hears you say are often two different things. It is no different with healthcare.

A patient came in and told the front desk he had a cough three weeks ago and that the cough went away but now he felt like his chest was congested and wanted to see if he had bronchitis or pneumonia. The person at the front desk wrote "cough" as his reason for coming in that day.

When the nurse called him to the exam room, she said, "You are here today for a cough?" He again explained the situation. She did not change his chart to reflect that he was there for chest congestion and *not* a cough.

I walked in and said, "So you are here for a cough?" By now the patient became angry and I can't blame him. No one seemed to get this right. In the next chapter, we will discuss ways you can get the personnel to repeat everything to you, so that such miscommunication does not cause you frustration.

Healthcare talks about teams and "patient-centered" medicine. This is all well and good, but it is window dressing on an opaque window. Did the healthcare system discuss their practices and procedures with the patients?

The Mayo Clinic is one of the best examples of patient-centered medicine and teamwork. Its culture of care holds high standards in team care for the patient. It seems to exemplify true patient-centered medicine, except when it doesn't. One patient traveled five hours to get to the Mayo Clinic, only to be told he was not there to see the doctor but to have his wound checked after he had had major surgery at this center. He could have done this at home, since he is a physician. He thought he was traveling back to speak to the surgeon about his operation. He would not have traveled five hours to have the nurse change his bandage. He had not known to ask the healthcare office why he had to return, nor had he told the healthcare office how far he had to travel to get to the Mayo Clinic, nor had he told the healthcare clinic his profession. He had not been asked to repeat his understanding of the next visit's goal. He never did see the surgeon again.

Asking the right questions is critical in finding the best doctor for you and the best services you need for recovery.

Mistake 3. Your Chart

Most of us spend more time figuring out what to wear every day than preparing to see our doctors. Your chart is one of the most critical and potentially deadliest parts of your healthcare. More and more patients are realizing they'd better keep a copy of their own medical chart.

Auto mechanics don't really need charts on our cars, but it is nice if they have them. Cell phone services don't really need charts, but they do like to keep a record of our calls, "for billing purposes." Banks not only keep charts on our finances but diligently send us monthly statements, so consumers can track their financial health. Should healthcare be different? We think not.

All your providers know how incomplete and wrong your charts are. If you had a healthcare chart that you had to reconcile monthly, you would soon see the dilemma your doctor is in when trying to figure out your safest treatment at the lowest cost for you. Why? Because charts are always wrong and incomplete.

To complicate matters more, your chart is made up of twenty-two parts with information that your provider must know and review before entering the exam room to see you. Every provider goes over all twenty-two parts if you are being admitted for surgery or hospitalization. The problem is that your chart is a mishmash of errors, inaccuracy, and disconnections and your providers know this.

One of my friends was admitted to the hospital for severe dehydration and abdominal pain. His liver test results were truly alarming, so the hospitalist (a stranger to this man's medical history) ordered an MRI (magnetic resonance imaging) of his liver. The liver showed two large masses and multiple nodules spread throughout his liver. He was told that, while the radiologist believed this was liver cancer, he believed the cancer came from another part of his body (it had metastasized). My friend's family notified me that their loved one had cancer and would soon get a biopsy but would need to be off his blood-thinning medication for forty-eight hours before the biopsy could be performed.

While this dear friend waited two long days in the hospital, fretting about the soon-to-be-confirmed cancer diagnosis, his sister remembered he had had a CT (computerized axial tomagraphy) scan of the abdomen two years prior and knew that record had to be somewhere. She finally obtained it and went straight to the hospitalist. The hospitalist sent it on to the radiologist, who consulted with other radiologists in his group. Collectively, they determined he was currently being misdiagnosed. The results of his recent MRI and his CT scan from two years before were identical. In other words, this was not cancer; what looked like tumors were hemangiomas (bloody areas in the liver), and there was no need to have alarmed the patient or performed a biopsy.

Let's look at the mental, emotional, physical, and financial impacts of the error that occurred because this man did not have his own set of records.

Mentally, he languished in the hospital for two days, stressed and worried about a cancer that was never to be. When he realized that this might be the end, he started to look at cancer treatment options and consider chemotherapy, which his hospitalist had already talked to him about. He got out his will and started to review it. Emotionally, his family was also in great distress.

Physically, he was not sleeping well, as the nurses were coming in to take his blood pressure every four hours, the phlebotomist was drawing his blood every morning at three thirty, and his bed squeaked every time he moved. He was hooked to an IV, which hurt his hand. So, between his lack of sleep, his exhaustion, and his incorrect diagnosis, he was heading toward depression.

Financially, he incurred the cost of staying in the hospital four extra days: two days because the hospital staff "forgot" to hold his blood-thinning medication before a biopsy could be performed. And two days so his sister could obtain that one missing piece of paper — the results of his two-year-old CT scan. (In the old days, his primary care provider would have known about this CT scan because he could have done "rounds" in the hospital himself. He also would have been able to connect with the radiologist right from the start and tell the radiologist about the abnormal liver finding.) This patient suffered a huge bill. And to think he went in for dehydration and needed only a bag of fluids, as nothing was found new or abnormal in his abdomen and the pain went away on its own!

The biggest mistake you can make as a patient is not to have your own complete set of records. Review them, share them, and have your doctor look at them for accuracy. Unless you master this one patient-driven directive, you will suffer at the hands of our healthcare system because your chart is always wrong.

Many times, when I am treating patients, the chart states that the patient is breastfeeding or pregnant. I look over at the exam table and there sits either a man or a woman in her nineties. Who puts this in your chart? I have no clue, but it can cost you your life; doctors who do not personally know you base their treatment decisions about your health and best practices on what your chart says.

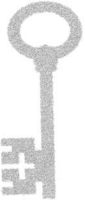

> Get all your records and keep them in a binder or obtain the Patient Best medical history binder at www.PatientBest.com. It is a medical record system written like your doctor's chart, to be reviewed by doctors in all specialties. Get your records, review them for accuracy, and keep them in that binder.

But my records are online. This is a major mistake a patient often makes. Your records online are not the same records your doctor reviews in the office. Specialists will often complain that your records are incomplete and they need the whole chart. Your records are always missing vital information. You do not know the twenty-two parts of your chart unless you have a specific binder or an advocate who can show you what this looks like.

But the nurse at the doctor's office always asks me, "Has anything changed in your chart since the last time you were here?" And most patients say no, though they do not have a clue what is in their charts. How can someone answer yes or no to a question they have no information about? We just do it out of habit, not realizing how critical our medical records are to our well-being. Surely, if our medical records are under such tight HIPAA (Health Insurance Portability and Accountability Act) regulation, the importance of these records warrants that their accuracy be confirmed by their owners.

At least ten times a week I will tell a patient that I cannot use a certain medication because it will interfere with one they are already taking (based on their chart). They tell me they are no longer taking that medication listed in their chart. This is an all-too-common error, especially important since certain medications are better or cost less than others.

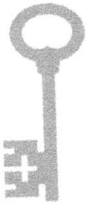

The person that escorts you to an examination room cannot take medications out of your chart or remove a misdiagnosis or resolved issue. It is usually only the provider who can do this, based on the policy of the clinic. Get a copy of your office visit record or have one mailed to you. Then read it and correct the mistakes. This book will show you how.

If the receptionist tells you that your office visit record is online, say that you want the record sent to you anyway. Not the whole chart, just today's office visit. Again, what is online and what is truly in your chart for all your doctors to see are two different things.

A client called her primary healthcare office and asked for a copy of her last office visit record. She was told it was online. She said she wanted it mailed to her instead. This healthcare system said they would mail it for $25.00 or she could get it online. She got it online.

Mistake 4. Misdiagnosis

Story after story comes out about mistakes like the one that Trisha Torrey tells on her website, www.TrishaTorrey.com. Trisha was told she had cancer, until she found out she didn't. No one wants to go through this. How do you protect yourself? Her story exemplifies the need for an advocate who knows that labs and pathology reports should have a second opinion.

Not all misdiagnoses have to be this severe. Many times patients are told they have an upper respiratory disease and given antibiotics, when in fact they have a virus and no antibiotics work on viruses. Is this harmful? Sure. The use of too many antibiotics can cause the development of antibiotic-resistant bacteria. What will we do when we don't have antibiotics to fight infection? Are we heading back to preantibiotic days due to massive ineffectiveness of the very antibiotics we created?

We see this a lot in women who come in for urinary tract infections, one of the most common reasons for an office visit. This is an infection found in the bladder. The urine is sent to the laboratory to confirm, with urine cultures, that bacteria are growing in the urine. When the cultures come back negative for growth, meaning there are no bacteria, patients are often given antibiotics anyway. Because the untrained patient does not request a copy of her urine culture, she has no idea that her discomfort may be from inflammation of the bladder and not infection. Years later, these same women are hospitalized when they do get infections because they need IV antibiotics to cure them, since they are victims of antibiotic-induced resistance to regular outpatient, oral antibiotics.

Understand that medicine is not an exact science. In his book *How Doctors Think*, Jerome Goodman gives examples of how pathology reports or x-rays can be misread, depending on the length of time the radiologist spends reading it or other factors.[1] It's always okay to get a second opinion. Many providers will respect this and be relieved that they are not missing something. "A second set of eyes" is what it's called in medicine. We will talk more about second opinions in our chapter on doctors' orders.

Mistake 5. Physical

Patients cannot go to the doctor, emergency room, or hospital without getting their bodies looked over. It's just the way it is. An auto mechanic cannot diagnosis your car trouble without seeing the car. Your bank cannot help you balance your account without knowing your account number. Some providers prefer that you take off your outerwear and put on a gown, so they can get a look at scars and moles or listen better to your heart, lungs, and abdomen. There is no right or wrong way here. Each provider is different and has his or her own set of preferences.

A patient came into a doctor's office and said she had "terrible pain" in her chest area. The doctor immediately ordered an EKG (electrocardiogram), which showed normal heart activity. The doctor then listened to her heart and lungs and examined her belly with the patient fully clothed. All seemed normal. The doctor surmised that the patient had gastroesophageal reflux (GERD), a stomach problem, and prescribed a certain medication. The patient returned two days later and said she still didn't feel better. This time the doctor *looked* at the patient's *skin* and saw a shingles rash across her left upper chest area. Misdiagnosis leads to time — and money — wasted.

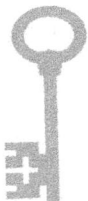

If your provider prefers you in a gown but the exam room is cold, then ask the back-office person for a blanket or bring a jacket with you. Most healthcare offices do not have control over the thermostats. The building maintenance personnel handle that.

Physical mistakes can range from missing the signs of a heart attack to missing a melanoma on the back of a patient's ear. Providers are taught to look, see, and smell. In the old days before glucose strips, my dad had to taste urine for sweetness (sugar) to diagnose a patient with diabetes. We have moved past that.

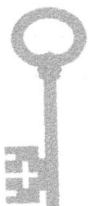

Each provider has her or his own way of examining patients. Some start at the top and some do not touch the patient at all. I once had a retired physician say, "What? You are actually examining my husband?" I did not understand the comment until she explained that many doctors do not touch the patient anymore but touch only the computer. This alarms me. Of concern is the patient who cannot move, whether a one-day-old infant or a hundred-year-old adult in a wheelchair. Doctors are taught to touch the skin, feel the warmth, get a pulse, see how the neck turns the head, observe movement of the chest with breathing and movement of limbs. Watching a baby sleep in a crib does not suffice for a true evaluation. During an examination, do not talk when your provider has the stethoscope on your body. We cannot hear a word you say. In fact, you sound like a bad speaker at a fast-food drive-though window. It's all mumbled. If the provider asks you a question, he or she will loosen the stethoscope from an ear to hear you speak. So please do *not* speak during your doctor's listening exam. And please, never, never speak when the provider has the stethoscope on your neck. The vibration is deafening. We can't pull the stethoscope away fast enough. Please help us out!

Most providers will watch you move about the room and even watch you get off the exam table. This is a way to assess your agility. Many providers will observe you moving down the hall or how you are sitting. Just know that this is part of your physical exam.

One emergency department I worked in had cameras outside its emergency room doors and others in the waiting room. They were there for protection and awareness. But we would often see patients come in walking perfectly normally and then double over and scream "back pain" and start writhing on the floor the minute they saw us coming. We would kindly help them up and get them to a waiting-room chair. They would ask to go ahead of everyone else due to their pain or beg us for pain medicines, but we would show them the cameras and they would stop begging and want to leave. Some of these patients would go down to the street corner, call 911, and ask the ambulance to take them to another emergency room. I hope they got the help they needed, and I'm sorry we couldn't help them.

Mistake 6. Social History

Social history is a big part of your chart. Remember those twenty-two parts of your chart? Well, this is one of them. In the old days, not only did my dad see you at weddings and funerals and know how much you drank or smoked, but if he did house calls, he also knew where and, more important, how you lived. That was the beauty of being a family practice doctor. All your habits were known to your provider.

How important is it for you to be honest with your provider? Let's say identical twins come into the office. They are in their sixties, female, and both have had the same cough for the past month. They grew up in a smoke-free home, but twin A started smoking at twenty-one and didn't quit. Twin B never smoked and was never around it.

The provider will examine each patient. Based on this information, the provider may order a chest x-ray on twin A but not on twin B. Since lung cancer cannot be heard, the provider may want to be sure twin A does not have it. But then twin B states that, while she never smoked, she did live in Kentucky all her adult life after moving away from home. Did anyone check her home for radon gas, a big cause of cancer, since this is a problem with limestone found throughout Kentucky? She says no, so now her provider may consider a chest x-ray to assess twin B for lung cancer. So social history can lead to a correct and early diagnosis. Catching diseases early on means a better outcome for all.

Our habits can be good or bad. You will ultimately decide how you want to live and how you can live. Your physician is your partner in your medical care and truly wants to stay on top of what is best for your situation. Social history — where you live, as well as your eating, drinking, smoking, and other habits — is important to your provider, so keep accurate records about your social life.

Your provider is not out to condemn your social habits. Yes, they will ask if you would like to advice on how to stop. But their focus is to keep you healthy and that means keeping an eye out for any early conditions so they can get you help sooner rather than later. If they don't know you smoke, they cannot order the right tests to discover lung cancer and head it off before it consumes you. If they don't know how much you drink, they can't keep an eye out for esophageal cancer or liver failure before it's too late. Also, if your liver or kidneys are damaged, they must be very careful about the medications and dosages they prescribe for you so they do not do more damage. Please tell your provider the truth. Medicine (not healthcare) is incredible in terms of new approaches and cures. We just need to get to know you sooner rather than later.

> One family practice doctor told me he had several patients who would book their appointments first thing in the morning so they didn't smell like smoke.

Mistake 7. Time

How is time a healthcare mistake or error? It is one of the biggest ones. It is important for you to understand that overworked doctors tend to make mistakes. If a doctor is overworked and exhausted and it's the end of the day, do you really want that physician doing surgery on you? According to Loehr and Schwartz in their book *The Full Power of Engagement*, energy is the key to focus, better outcomes, and positive interactions.[2] When fatigue sets in, what kind of care are you getting? Setting an appointment at the right time of the day or month is the key to better outcomes in medical care.

Years ago, providers could spend all the time they wanted getting to know you and visiting with you. Big-business healthcare today expects providers to see a patient in ten to fifteen minutes. This puts impossible pressure on physicians and patients, and therefore the waiting room becomes jammed up. In our healthcare system, big business sees time as money, and most providers are paid according to the number of patients they see in minutes, not the number of minutes spent with a patient. In the sales world, it's called commission. In the healthcare world, it's called RVUs (Relative Value Units). The number of RVUs a provider gets out of your office visit, surgery, or hospital stay will determine what that provider gets in her or his paycheck.

Many new doctors work for two or three years in clinics before they can build up their practices. During this time, they are on salary. The production, or number of patients they see, can sometimes determine what their commission structure will be. Once on full "commission," they must see more patients to get paid. The problem is that you are an individual and different from every other patient. Slow the doctor down with your concerns and your questions or find yourself a direct primary care or private practice doctor.

Midlevel providers, on the other hand, are usually paid a flat hourly wage, but they too can get "bonuses" based on their billing. This incentivizes your providers to see more patients and do more in terms of procedures and office visits.

We will talk more about types of questions you need to ask and satisfactory answers you should hear when you are racing against time and vying for your provider's attention in a ten-minute office visit.

Mistake 8. Abandonment

One of the worst disasters in healthcare can occur in the form of abandonment. This healthcare error is often a result of the discontinuity between and among healthcare professionals. Failure to get your reports can cost you your life. Anytime you, the patient, get an order for labs, a biopsy, or an imaging study like an x-ray, MRI, bone density scan, CT scan, or even dental x-rays, you must always request a report be sent to your home. You want to make sure you get a copy, so you can go over it with the ordering provider. There are no checks and balance to be sure every image or lab is followed up with a report. We will talk more about going over reports in chapter 9 on doctors' orders.

One patient was told by her gynecologist that she needed a CT scan of her uterus to rule out uterine cancer. The office told her that if she didn't hear anything, then it was normal. The report came back positive for cancer, but no one called the patient. For over a year, she didn't know she had this cancer. When she went to an urgent clinic for a cough, the doctor took the time to review her chart and saw the cancer report. The doctor asked her about it and the patient almost fainted. She had no idea she had cancer. Always, 100 percent of the time, get a copy of your results and go over them with your doctor.

Contrast the above patient with this one. One young woman had seven different blood tests done. She knew to always get results back. When she requested a copy of her labs be sent to her home, she received only four results. She called the ordering doctor's office and they couldn't find the other three. The only proof she had that these labs were done was her bill for all seven labs. So the ordering doctor's staff started to hunt down the results through the lab service. They finally found them and sent them to her after her doctor looked at them. Loosing results is a common occurrence, as healthcare has no checks and balances to see if reports actually get back to the ordering doctor.

Many times your provider is looking for your last labs or imaging study but can't find it. Where did you have the test done? When did you get the test completed?

All providers know that when patients tell us, "Oh, I have my charts online," terror strikes us and we mentally roll our eyes. Why? Because we know your chart "online" is incomplete and you are probably missing information, or worse, it's wrong. You don't think so? Ask for your "doctor's chart" and see how much missing information and wrong information it has about you. When you start collecting the twenty-two sections of your chart, you will see the inaccuracies.

Another type of abandonment is found at the point of "hospital discharge." Some patients used to be sent home from the hospital by taxi with no family support at home. This began to show up as a massive problem when patients were returning to the hospital within thirty days of being discharged, for the same or worse problems.

Insurance companies took notice and denied payment for these returning visits, so hospitals started looking at ways to find support systems for these patients, so they would get the home care and support they needed in order to get better. Many times a hospital will tell a patient to follow up with their primary care provider within ten days of a hospital discharge, but the problem is that these patients cannot get in to see their primary care providers for months afterward.

Hospitals began losing billions of dollars for mishandling patients and now employ social workers and patient navigators to get support systems in place for patients so they don't "bounce back." Some discharge plans will send a patient to a "nursing home" for thirty days so they don't bounce back. Sending a patient home without proper care and follow-up with medical providers is a type of abandonment that must stop. Patient advocates are invaluable to their clients when they are discharged.

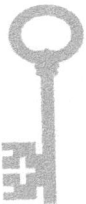

Get your plans in place ahead of time. Get home health, a physical therapist, and other home care providers lined up the minute you are admitted to the hospital. Some hospitals have their own home health service. Just make sure it's the best service for you. Not all services are the same. If you have a patient advocate, the advocate will know the best providers in your community and you will know the right questions to ask to get the best one for you.

Here is a recent example of hospital systems still failing. A patient entered the hospital with alcohol poisoning. The social worker was contacted to see the patient and discuss his drinking habits. She visited the patient within twelve hours of admission. He was still under the influence of alcohol and heavy medical sedation. He slept through her visit as she rambled on about alcohol rehabilitation. Five days later, the patient was stable enough to return home. The social worker was asked by the family what interventions were available and, now that the patient was coherent, whether she could please revisit him and discuss options. She told the family that she was already discharged from the case. She had "checked the box" stating that she spoke to him even though he slept through her one-sided conversation. Abandonment. So the patient will return, and the hospital will pay for this in poor ratings and financial loss while the family suffers emotional, physical, and mental anguish over their loved one. This was not the social worker's fault. She had over thirty-five cases to work on and her administration did not seem to hear her anguish.

Mistake 9. Emotional

Healthcare mistakes due to emotional crisis are very common. In 1990, Dr. Harold P. Freeman of the Freeman Patient Navigation Institute saw the devastation wrought by breast cancer on women in Harlem, New York, and decided to help these women get through the confusion and fear they experienced in their encounters with healthcare. This was the actual beginning of health or patient advocacy as a vocation.[3]

There is a common phenomenon called shock diagnosis syndrome. This occurs when a patient is given a devastating diagnosis and does not hear another word the doctor says. Because this occurs, many physicians will call in the family when such a diagnosis must be discussed. Still, the emotional trauma trumps listening skills. Conversation ceases. Physician's orders, the plan of treatment, and actions to be taken should not be discussed at this time. When meeting with your doctor to discuss a serious diagnosis, take someone with you who can take notes. Many patients will bring their patient advocate with them as well as their family.

Physicians and their medical teams are all under emotional stress as well. A survey within one very large hospital asked the medical team how they felt about their work. Here's an example of their emotional plight:

> "I began to feel like an easily replaceable cog in the health-care machine. With the [enforcement] of EHRs, I had to spend more time as a scribe. One night a child I was treating had a seizure and I couldn't get the medicine to enable them to breathe because their chart wasn't in the system yet. This kid was fixing to die and I, the doctor, couldn't get the medicine. It was demoralizing." – Amy Baxter, MD[4]

What Are the Causes of Burnout in Family Physicians?

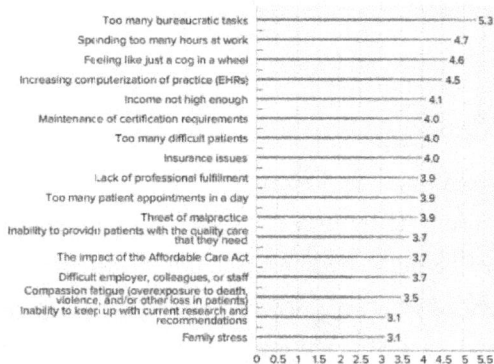

Too many bureaucratic tasks	5.3
Spending too many hours at work	4.7
Feeling like just a cog in a wheel	4.6
Increasing computerization of practice (EHRs)	4.5
Income not high enough	4.1
Maintenance of certification requirements	4.0
Too many difficult patients	4.0
Insurance issues	4.0
Lack of professional fulfillment	3.9
Too many patient appointments in a day	3.9
Threat of malpractice	3.9
Inability to provide patients with the quality care that they need	3.7
The impact of the Affordable Care Act	3.7
Difficult employer, colleagues, or staff	3.7
Compassion fatigue (overexposure to death, violence, and/or other loss in patients)	3.5
Inability to keep up with current research and recommendations	3.1
Family stress	3.1

0 0.5 1 1.5 2 2.5 3 3.5 4 4.5 5 5.5

What causes burnout in family physicians? (https://www.medscape.com/features/slideshow/lifestyle/2017 family-medicine#page=4)

Physicians are called upon to do too much but not even given the authority to decide what is best for their practice. Because bureaucracy decides how doctors will treat patients, how many they will see, and how they will chart, patients are left out of the care plan.

Mistake 10. Neglect

Neglect is a two-sided indifference. Patients often ignore their health problems until they are worse. Healthcare ignores patients. Doctors who cry out for help, to spend more time with patients, are also ignored by healthcare. And then, in turn, patients ignore the poor service they get. We understand this is a very real result of capitalism within healthcare. It also means that the patient may ignore treatment orders, labs, and medical bills. Let's look at how healthcare neglects the patient.

Hospitalists are revenue generators, which means the providers do not have the time they need to sit with you and your family and discuss what is truly going on. The hospitalist usually comes in when you, the patient, are sleeping (Is this on purpose?) and wakes you out of whatever drug-induced coma you may be in to tell you what is going on. Naturally, as a patient, you cannot remember anything to tell your family, who are not there at the time. Did that doctor come in? Or was I dreaming?

The rest of the hospital staff do not generate revenue, so they must squeeze as many order completions into an hour as they can. Because healthcare is overworking its staff of registered nurses (RNs), certified nursing assistants (CNAs), and social workers, there is no time to waste. Therefore, they give you a call button and you think, I push this and the RN will come running. Not so fast. The RN is overworked. Someone may show up thirty minutes after you get out of the bed and use the restroom. But wait, you were told not to get up out of bed. Too late. It is what patients do when they are neglected.

Okay, worse. You fall. Then risk management (the big legal gurus) microscope the scenario. Why did you fall? Why didn't the nurse come in time? Oh, the RN was busy saving another patient's life. "No excuse," says the risk management. The RN is at fault and will be "written up."

Let's talk about healthcare nutrition. What? That's when they dump cold, inedible food on a tray and leave it in your room. Where is it left? Across the room so you can't reach it. Okay, so hit that call button again. See if anyone moves the tray for you. Let's get up and get the tray. Fall risk. And so the cycle goes.

Let's talk about getting out of the hospital. Who takes care of you, the patient, when you return home? Medical practice dictates that you cannot be sent home in a cab, paid private driver service, or bus anymore. You must have a family member with you to keep track of you so you don't bounce back into the hospital. Remember, the hospital gets fined big-time if you bounce back within thirty days. Some states have legislation that mandates that hospitals can't send you home without support. Why? Because big-business healthcare wanted your bed for someone else and your stay was good for only a certain number of days before your insurance stopped paying, so off you went!

Another form of neglect: Your healthcare office will not call you back. You have questions. Healthcare does not allow their physicians to call you back. Physicians are seeing thirty to forty patients in a day, generating revenue, reviewing labs and radiology reports, following up on insurance bills, and charting. Remember, a third of a doctor's day is spent charting. That's healthcare. A nurse or some other employee must call you back. That can take days because of the numerous people and systems healthcare has snuck in between you and your doctor.

Another type of neglect occurs when the pharmacist has a question for your doctor about your medication. Maybe it has an interaction with another drug you are taking. Why didn't the doctor notice this? Because your chart, which the doctor is using as a guide, is wrong. It didn't have that drug on there. So you and the other hundreds of patients will wait several days before the doctor and staff can call the pharmacist back, and then you can get your medication. Neglect.

You call your physician because you have a cold and need to be seen today. The office staff says they can get you in six weeks from now. You are mad at your doctor (not the healthcare system), so you head off to an urgent care facility and get treated there. What you need to know is that your doctor has no idea you even called. In fact, your doctors have no clue how many patients are being turned away on a daily basis. Big-business healthcare is telling your doctor to see thirty and more patients a day, and there is no room for "same-day visits." And we, as patients, are neglecting the fact that this is poor service. Why do we accept it? How do we stop accepting poor service? Ask the right questions.

Mistake 11. Financial

If healthcare is going to survive it must make money. Any business must. In fact, it is investors who take the risk and therefore expect a return on their investment. The healthcare system is no different. Let's look at how the revenue in healthcare is generated. There are three main considerations.

1. Providers are the main revenue generators for their employers.
2. Patients do not scrutinize their medical bills.
3. Healthcare insurance companies have the power to deny or pay medical bills.

Companies stay in business in direct relation to the amount of capital they have. Knowing this, we have to think about who the income producers are in the health system. Medical orders and services are written by doctors. This means that, unless the hospital has a doctor, nurse practitioner, or physician assistant to write the order, no revenue is generated. The orders they write support hundreds of employees.

Let's say you have two doctors. One writes orders for labs, an X-ray, and an office visit and asks you to return in three months. The other doctor just charges you for today's office visit. The first doctor generated lab and x-ray revenue and ensured future revenue. Lab fees can help pay for the nurse, call center, receptionist, billing clerk, coder, administrator, phlebotomist, test tube, and lab tech. The same with the x-ray order.

The second doctor did no such thing. Orders generate revenue. Period.

Healthcare has one resource to generate its revenue — the doctor, physician assistant, or nurse practitioner. That's it. These three professionals bring in the revenue. Without an order, no revenue is generated and no one gets income.

Physicians are well aware of the revenue they must generate in order to keep a clinic open and afloat. When insurance is involved, the costs of electronic medical records can be in the millions, in addition to malpractice insurance, medical equipment, utilities for the clinic, and more. But many patients do not realize that it is the ordering provider that has to bring in that revenue.

I have worked in multiple clinics but never as much as in the one where I was the single provider and my patient visits and orders had to support fourteen salaries. As I looked around the clinic, I realized I had two receptionists at the front desk. One supervisor for them, three nurses, one x-ray technician, one supervisor for the back-office personnel, one billing coder, one billing insurance person, one human resources person, and two cleaning service persons.

Then there was my salary. No income could be generated without me. By seeing the patient and charging for the office visit, I generated one stream of revenue.

If providers across the country stopped writing orders for one day, would it crash their employers' revenue streams? It might. Instead of a walk-out, it would be a "write-out." No orders. Period. All prescriptions halted. Drugstores would tremble; hospitals would lay people off.

But hospitals charge for their hospital rooms. True, but not enough revenue is generated. Intravenous fluids, medication orders, imaging studies, and labs every twenty-four hours all bring in the revenue necessary to keep the hospital afloat. Now you understand why one-third of all labs are unnecessary every year, accounting for $200 billion in wasted money but not wasted revenue for the employer.[5]

Now let's talk about the patient's side of cost. Whew! There's nothing like medical billing. First and foremost, you want to understand that medical costs are the biggest cause of bankruptcy in America today. Patients cannot pay these exorbitant fees but do not realize they have the right to hire a patient advocate who specializes in getting the bill corrected. The average bill is reduced by 70 percent. Medical bills go through multiple systems before they are generated. The coder evaluates the doctor's bill to see whether it is coded correctly or whether any charges are left on the table. Once the bill is confirmed it goes to the billing clerk, who reviews it and sends it to the correct insurance company. The insurance company decides what they will pay or not pay. Then it goes to their biller to generate a "This is not a bill" statement. Then it goes back to the provider, who will send out the provider's portion of the bill to you. It is not checked for accuracy but for revenue generation. The fine print in your insurance policy dictates that they do not have to pay. They have to the power to decide what they can deny. Just trust me on this.

But take heart. You're not the only one who doesn't get coverage. Doctors and other healthcare providers bill your insurance company. The insurance company may say no for no reason at all. They can make up a reason. Maybe they took their cue from the airlines business. Ever notice how airlines just cancel a flight for the heck of it? You go up to the counter and ask why your flight was cancelled and they read off the screen, "Today is Tuesday so we will tell all passengers the flight has been cancelled due to mechanical failure." And your plane changes gates and takes off in another direction. Or maybe they say it's "due to weather," although all the other planes are flying out and the skies tell you a different story. Likewise, insurance companies will say no for any reason they choose. After all, how can your monthly premium pay for that gargantuan operation? Who keeps the largest buildings? The insurance companies.

While insurance companies employ thousands of people, and the above picture is only one of many corporate headquarters Blue Cross / Blue Shield has, people would be out jobs if patients started refusing unnecessary tests or began scrutinizing their bills.

Medical bills are *always* wrong, and we will look this in chapter 11.

Mistake 12. Unqualified Patients

How can a patient be unqualified? Easily. One example is the hospital patient who is woken at five a.m. by the staff to take another sleeping pill. The patient was sleeping just fine. Ten minutes later, the same patient is woken to get blood from a vein. Ten minutes later a hospitalist walks in to tell the drugged patient that he or she is going home today. This is an unqualified patient, because the patient is sleeping.

Drugs "unqualify" patients all the time. Pain medications are wonder drugs but can mentally derange a patient. This patient is not qualified to make choices for her- or himself. The patient rights violated in this case are informed consent and shared decision making.

Another unqualified patient is the one who was just told he or she has cancer. That's it. That's all the patient heard. No other words were heard after the big C. So the patient is not qualified to follow any directions after that. Next thing you know, you the patient are headed to another appointment and still don't know why or where you are going. You are clueless as to tests and events that will follow. You are, in this case, an unqualified patient. But healthcare says your provider must see more patients in a day and so must get these patients out of the office as fast as possible.

Let's talk about the patient whose mental capacity is limited but who is able to function on a day-to-day basis if her or his day is stabilized. This is the person who is taken to the ER and has no clue or comprehension of what's happening. Family can't get there fast enough. The patient's chart is incomplete, so no staff member knows that this patient is diagnosed with mental disabilities. What happens? The patient sits in bed saying, "I'm fine" every time a doctor comes in. The staff has no clue otherwise.

An emergency room physician was seeing a patient who was obviously legally blind. She carried the white cane and wore dark glasses, and she usually had her patient advocate with her on medical visits, but not on this emergency visit. Her ER doctor discharged her and told her to walk thirty minutes a day for better health and to follow up with her primary care provider.

She then came in to see me for her follow-up appointment. As I was reviewing her chart, I saw no mention of her eyesight. Imagine my surprise when I entered the room; I was disheartened to know that no one had put this information in her chart. In fact, her ER chart was a preworded template. It mentioned her eyesight as normal. Had the ER provider taken the time to address her eyesight, then discussion of how to walk safely should have been addressed.

And then there's the patient with no insurance. Healthcare systems like to be paid. While all emergency rooms must take the uninsured, outpatient medical practices are not required to do so. So you call and say you would like to establish care with a certain PCP (primary care provider). Healthcare tells the office staff to say, "Please send us your medical records so we can review them." What they are actually saying is, "Please send us your medical records so we can see what kind of insurance you have and whether it pays on a regular basis."

Mistake 13. Noncompliant Patients

This is a big one. This is the patient who does not follow through on the doctor's orders. There are usually many options for treatment. Some patients only get one option, depending on the questions they ask. Other patients find the instructions too complicated, costly, or tiresome.

Obesity is rampant in America but so are the quick and easy processed foods and sodas sold on every street corner.

My friend Denise Pancyrz is a diabetes reversal coach and an author. Her book *The Virgin Diabetic* flies off the shelf because it gives a natural alternative to diabetic recovery. Through holistic lifestyle coaching, Denise takes customization and personalization to a new level. Her clients' successes lie in several areas within a person's life — stress, rest, how to incorporate activity without going to the gym (unless you want to), education on the foods that heal diabetes, how to set up your kitchen, grocery shopping, and how to dine at your favorite restaurants without sabotaging yourself.

The service is very personalized, and her ability to ferret out the preservatives, hidden sugars, and added ingredients in American food gives her clients a roadmap to the foods that cause their sugars to increase. Clients learn the secret to stop counting carbs and still achieve remarkable A1c (glycated hemoglobin, which tells you how much sugar is attached to the blood proteins) levels. While doctors will treat diabetes with diet and exercise, many Americans know this is difficult, since there is a fast-food restaurant or coffee shop on every corner in America. What is a patient to do? The next trip to the doctor finds the patient on medication for life. This is the option Denise was given in her personal story; she chose otherwise. Is she compliant? Yes, but by making her own choice. She saw a better way and embraced recovery successfully. Denise learned it's not about eliminating foods, which is the norm in diabetes classes. Now she teaches others to do the same.

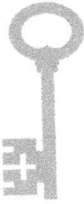

Tell your doctor what your habits are and what you struggle with. Doctors, nurses, and physician assistants are truly there to help you, not judge you. Let's say you drink six to ten carbonated beverages (sodas) a day. This not only rots your stomach lining but also gives you indigestion and bloating. Your doctor can't get you to stop drinking sodas, or maybe your chart doesn't indicate that you do, and you are not about ready to mention this. So you doctor prescribes medications for your condition. You don't get better. Of course, you won't. You are not stopping the cause. Now your doctor is puzzled. Maybe there is "something else" going on. Concern sets in, so your doctor sends you to a "specialist" who will look inside your belly to see what the problem is. Okay, so off your go to the gastroenterologist, who has you swallow a camera and looks down your throat. Oh, wait. No soda there. Why? Because you couldn't eat or drink since midnight the night before. Hmmm. Lots of inflamed stomach tissue, though. Okay, no cancer. Let's try more medications. (Did I mention that all medications have side effects?)

Medical errors follow: now your throat hurts because of the endoscope, your wallet hurts because there was a huge co-pay for the specialist (the pathologist has a bill, too), your time going and coming to and from the specialist has been wasted, and there are still no answers except "Everything looks pretty normal." You should have just told your doctor how many sodas you drank a day.

Mistake 14. Failed Care Coordination

The last, but surely not the least common, medical error in healthcare today is failed care coordination. In fact, one study shows that only seven percent of a hospital's patients were fully care coordinated from hospital to home care. Thirty percent had some care coordination.[6] Patient advocates are critical to care coordination. Their success lies in the fact that they stay focused on you, the patient. They do not have overloaded caseloads of patients to push out of the hospital, take to the doctor, or organize home health for. They are your personal, customized navigators, who oversee the best care services in town for you.

Failed care coordination weaves itself into every line of healthcare. Here are some examples:

→ The patient receives a refund (for something she never should have been billed for in the first place) thirteen months after her visit.

→ The doctor orders a medication not on the patient's list of covered medications.

→ You talk to a call center and are told the convenient care center can see you. But when you arrive you are told there is no CT scanner and you need to go to the ER.

→ Your family doctor sends you to a "specialist" and that doctor has no clue why the doctor sent you. Your co-pay? $60.00

→ The patient checks in at the kiosk and is told to swipe his or her credit card for $225, but is given no explanation. The receptionist says to ignore it and just wait for a bill. Why even bother with a kiosk? Because patients do not ask the right questions and there is no coordination.

→ The doctor is told you are visiting today for a "terminitis of the global lobe," but you are really there for a "dermatitis of the lower leg." Remember, the front desk clerk does not have a medical background. Therefore, you should ask the front-desk clerk to please read back what they wrote you are there for.

CHAPTER 4

The Players

Before we can talk about the system, we have to go over a few terms and identify the players. There are now many professionals in the system and we cannot begin to list them all. We will discuss the major ones, and when you come across others, you can always ask them what their role is.

The PCP. The what? The primary care provider is the main family practice doctor. Every patient — young, old, or in-between — needs a primary care provider, also known as your main doctor. This is your go-to medical partner. This is the most important player on your medical field. You do not want to launch until you have a "quarterback" to help you get through any medical dilemma.

Now let's talk about what this PCP looks like. There are four main types of PCP, and you should know the differences and similarities. The MD is the doctor of medicine. Another type of physician holds a DO, doctor of osteopathic medicine. The third is the physician assistant, who is supervised by a physician (MD or DO) and can practice alone or in a practice with the physician. The fourth PCP you might see is the nurse practitioner. Nurse practitioners may or may not need a supervising physician, depending on what the laws are in their particular state and what their specialty is. All four providers can be found in all specialties, as well as in clinics and hospitals. Nurse practitioners and physician assistants can treat you, write prescriptions, admit you to the hospital, order labs and imaging studies, or perform surgery. To you, the patient, there should be no difference between these professions. Choose whomever you are most comfortable with.

For those of you who want to know more details about the background educational requirements of the different types of provider, here you go. The latter two professions have spent fewer years in training. Every state regulates these four professions. All four professionals are collectively called "providers" in today's medical world.

Physician assistants and nurse practitioners are sometimes referred to as "midlevels" or "advanced providers." Their training differs. Physician assistant schools require their applicants to have a bachelor's degree from a four-year accredited school. They then give up two to three years of their lives to study medicine. They attend PA school full-time. Their first year(s) are spent in classroom study. These students are required to dissect a cadaver along with medical students and take organic chemistry. They are trained in the medical model, exactly like physicians. Their last years of study are spent in clinical practice. Their clinical study is under the supervision of physicians. They will typically spend two months in family practice and then one month in each of the following: hospitalist work, internal medicine, surgery, pediatrics, obstetrics and gynecology, psychiatry, emergency room medicine, and specialized areas of interest. Every school has variations in the clinical studies, but these are the prerequisites for graduation. They will have at least two thousand hours of clinical study and practice before they graduate.

The nurse practitioner requirements are that an applicant must be a nurse with a bachelor's degree in nursing or its equivalent and complete a doctor of nursing program. These courses may be online. Dissecting cadavers is not a requirement. Clinical rotations must be at least six hundred hours in the area of interest: psychiatry, pediatrics, family medicine, or obstetrics and gynecology. They can work full-time while studying to become a doctor of nursing practice.

Physician assistants are usually called by their first name, as they hold a master's degree in physician assistant studies. Nurse practitioners may use the term "doctor," as they hold a doctor of nursing practice degree.

Both midlevels are focused on returning you to good health and tending to your concerns and safety. You may choose to have any one of these four as your primary care provider. The key is that you trust the person to do what is best for you.

Now that you have established a PCP (see, you are already learning the lingo), it is important to understand that all your healthcare should originate from this provider's office. What is meant by that? Well, think about it. When you visit your PCP, you may leave with a set of orders: medicines and such medical services as physical therapy, surgery, medical equipment, or even the services of another provider. Think of your PCP as the one medical person whose job is to see the whole picture of you and your health. He or she is the one you can tell your deep, dark secrets to. He or she is there for you as the two of you grow old together. He or she will trust you to always tell the truth, so that your PCP can better know you and watch out for any stones that may get thrown into your healthcare path. He or she also knows whom to send you to when you need something beyond his or her scope of practice.

We mentioned the role of the certified patient advocate, in chapter 1. These men and women have passed a national exam written by the Patient Advocate Certification Board in ethics, scope of practice, and law in order to become certified. They can be generalists or specialists. Generalists will serve your needs in many capacities and guide you through the healthcare system smoothly. Examples of certified patient advocate specialties are medical billing (getting your bills reduced), hospitalizations (care, safety, and infection control), country (locating the best physicians and services in the country), dementia care (helping families cope and get the needed resources), and transitions.

For example, you may find yourself needing to move to a community housing or assisted living facility. Which is best for you? The certified patient advocate will not only help you find the perfect place but also find the right realtor and the right person to help you take the precious things you want and dispose of the rest, and coordinate the move so that you do not need to do a thing. Let's look at other similar roles within the healthcare system.

A patient navigator is someone who is employed by a large healthcare system. They will help patients get the care they need, but their hands are typically tied in terms of how much they can help someone because of the workload they carry. One patient navigator told me she saw over 950 clients in a year.

When you are discharged from the hospital, you will have a discharge person. The hospital employs these people to get you discharged, finding a suitable place to send you if you cannot go home. This person is typically overloaded as well. While they do the same or similar functions as patient navigators, both positions terminate their relationship with the patient when the patient leaves the facility. A certified patient advocate will keep working with the patient no matter where they seek healthcare, as their focus is on the patient, not the advocate's employer.

Many facilities and state laws refer to "patient advocate" using the term loosely. This makes it very confusing to most of us. To be sure you are working with the right person, ask whether the person owns his or her own practice and whether you will pay this advocate directly.

There are many concepts of what patient advocates are and what they do.

A patient asked her provider for a referral to have her knee replaced. Her PCP gave her a name. The patient did some research and found this orthopedic surgeon did not have the best reputation for replacing knees. At least that's what her friends told her. That was okay. She asked around until she found a patient advocate. The advocate knew exactly who had the best outcomes, shortest recovery times, and fewest infections. How? Anesthesiologists always know what goes on in the surgery rooms. Patient advocates know this and seek out friendships with all the knowledgeable workers in their respective fields of expertise in healthcare. The patient called her PCP, who was more than happy to accommodate her request for this new referral, and learned an interesting lesson from this experience. When the newly referred orthopedic surgeon called her PCP to thank her for referring a patient and to give her all the follow-up information on how well the patient did, the PCP decided to switch her referrals to this new orthopedist. So this is a two-way street. Do not think your doctors don't learn from you. In my experience, I have seen patients educating their physicians on multiple issues. Physicians appreciate the time you take to do your homework, too. In my own practice, my network of referrals for highly specialized medicine comes from patients who have traveled all over the world to get the best of the best practitioners to take care of the riskiest surgeries and rarest diseases.

Next, remember what I said earlier — that most people spend more time deciding what to wear in the morning than preparing for their doctor's visit. "What, I have to prepare? For what?" One of many secrets all patients have to understand is that healthcare (notice that I didn't say medical) delivery is an art all to itself. There are certain rules that have to be followed in order to get you in and out of the provider's office in a timely manner. "Timely?" you say. "I spend hours waiting for my appointments. Why can't providers be on time?"

Okay, lesson two: Providers could be on time if all their patients were trained like a well-tuned marching band to know the exact steps that have to occur with every provider's office visit.

So let's start part 2 of this book with the most important event of all: the office visit.

Your Steps to 5-Star Healthcare

CHAPTER 5

Your Office Visit

Before Your Visit

Step 1. Calling to Make the Appointment

You call the provider's office to set up an appointment. Well, wait a minute. Are you really calling the office or are you calling a call center somewhere in Walla Walla, Washington? How do you know? Are you speaking to someone who knows the professional medical jargon or are you speaking to someone who has no clue what a nasal polyp is? (A growth in the nose.) Maybe the person thinks you said, "Basil dollop" and were making Italian sauce and meatballs. How do we providers know this happens? Because these are the messages we see every day. "Patient wants a basil dollop." We have no clue why you are coming into the office for this. Nothing surprises us anymore.

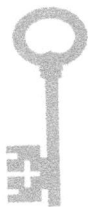

When you call to make an appointment, you will ask who the person is you are speaking to and write down the person's name and position. Ask if the person is medically trained. Now you can give your message. But you are not done. Before you get off the phone, ask the person to *read* the message back to you. You will be shocked at all the missing pieces.

A patient called in to say the new medicine she was taking for her high blood pressure was giving her diarrhea. She wanted another medicine called in that wouldn't give her this problem. The message the provider got on her computer was "Patient now has diarrhea." So the provider called in a medicine for diarrhea. Patient picked up her second medicine and assumed it was the new medicine for her high blood pressure (without the side effect of diarrhea) so she stopped taking the first medicine and took only the second one. Her blood pressure was not controlled, and she had to return to the provider's office a week later to see why she was now constipated and the "blood pressure" medicine wasn't working. *In addition*, she had to pay another office visit co-pay.

Can you see why it is so important to always have the message read back to you?

Step 2. Setting up the Appointment

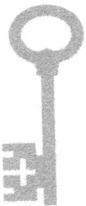

When setting up appointments, it is best to schedule them first thing in the morning or be the first patient in the afternoon. Many patients know that this will get you in and out faster, so you may be hard-pressed to find a date when the office can accommodate you. We will talk more about this later as you learn all the steps to building a relationship with the office staff and the providers.

Also, try to never schedule your appointment on a Monday, a Friday, the day before or after a holiday, or the day before or after your PCP is on vacation. These are the most heavily scheduled days and the office is the busiest during these times. Oh, and don't forget the end of the year, too. Patients who have met their deductible start filling their days with doctor's appointments to get everything they need done before a new year and new deductibles kick in.

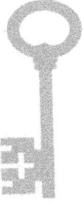

If you cannot get in to see your PCP, ask to see if a physician assistant or nurse practitioner can see you. Many times I was seeing "same-day visits," which are patients who want to be seen on the day they call; many times the doctor would stop in to say hello to the patient. If I had any questions, I could always ask the doctor. This is one of the greatest services your doctor can offer you — same day visits. My schedule was empty every morning, and by ten a.m. I would be booked with thirty to thirty-five patients who needed to be seen immediately. If your doctor's practice does not offer this, then encourage them to hire a midlevel for same-day visits. If your doctor's office cannot get you in, then you will have to go to an urgent care clinic, wait longer, pay more, and be seen by someone who does not know you or your medical history. This is a setup for failure.

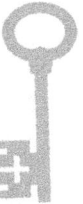

Ask how long your appointment is for. You want to honor the provider's time and try to be in and out in the time that has been allotted for you. Your doctor will wish she or he had a thousand patients like you.

Okay, now let's move on to the office visit preparation.

Step 3. Preparing for the Office Visit

If this is the first time you are seeing a certain physician or healthcare facility, then arrive twenty to thirty minutes early. You are going to fill out paperwork. In some cases, you will be handed a tablet and asked to read everything and sign with your finger. Isn't technology great?

Make sure your own set of medical records is up to date and complete with all your information. Bring your own medical history book with you. If you do not have one, then build one and get it together as soon as possible. We have already seen that records are wrong. You need your own set of personal records. A good medical history binder will save life, money, and time over and over again. If you need a complete binder with all twenty-two parts and written like a doctor's chart, see www.PatientBest.com/binder for more information. *Chief complaint* (CC) is the name providers use for the reason you are seeing them. Usually you come in with more than one complaint, but we still want to know the chief complaint. Let's say your chief complaint is a cough you would like the PCP to look at. But when you get the office, you remember that you have had dizziness lately and would like to ask about that. Remember when we talked about why you have to wait so long in the doctor's office? Well, now that patient behind you is going to have to wait because you just added another complaint to your list. That's okay though, because I am going to show you how you are going to get in and out of the provider's office quickly.

Before you go to the office visit, you are going to have all this information written down. Remember that your chart is different from an office visit record. Your chart is huge and contains twenty-two parts. "Today's Office Visit" contains only one — today's office visit.

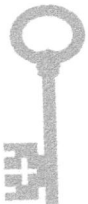

You are going to write down on a paper all your complaints. No, start with your chief complaint. You are going to use the same method every doctor uses to discern the history behind this complaint. This method is called OLD CARTS. This is an ordered method for obtaining the information your doctor must have in order to get paid by your insurance company.

So you are going to be the exceptional patient that every doctor loves, because you have OLD CARTS completed for every complaint.

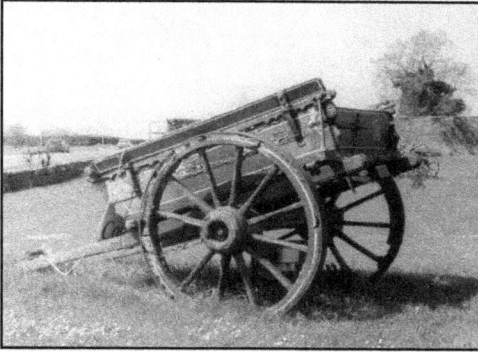
Old Carts

So, what does OLD CARTS mean?

O = Onset. When did the symptoms start?

L = Location. Where is the pain, cough, headache, weakness, rash, etc.?

D = Duration. When it starts, how long does it last? Does the pain wax and wane? Does the cough start and not stop? Does the headache come and go? How often are you going to the bathroom?

C = Characteristic. Describe what it feels or looks like. For example, is the pain sharp, burning, dull, aching? Is the rash itching, painful? Is the cough productive or not productive? Is the urine red, dark, burning, or frequent?

A = Aggravating. What makes these symptoms worse? Heat? Cold? Write down the *names* of any over-the-counter (OTC) medicines you have already tried.

A patient comes in for a rash and says she tried an over-the-counter cream that her pharmacist said might help, but it hasn't. She does not know the name of the cream she tried. Her provider is at a loss to try her on any new medications for the rash unless he knows the one she has already tried. Why? Because what he selects might be similar to the cream she has already tried. She would be wasting her time and money on something that won't work. Her provider is more than happy to help her but needs to know all the medicines she has tried.

R = Relieving factors. What makes the pain better? Heat? Cold? Did acetaminophen or ibuprofen help? Did you eat something that made your belly pain better or worse? (R could also stand for "Radiates": Does the pain radiate to another part of your body?)

T = Timing. Does the pain get better at night or during the day? How about the urinary tract infection — better or worse before or after a meal? Does lying down at night make your cough worse or better? Are you coughing worse at work or at home?

S = Other Symptoms related to your complaint. For example, you have a cough, but do you also have a temperature with it? What about nausea or vomiting? Do you have a rash? You sprained your ankle; do you have previous injury to that same ankle? When you walk on it, does it hurt your back? Do you have numbness or tingling? What other signs are you having with your chief complaint and all the others?

Here's what your paper will look like:

TODAY'S OFFICE VISIT GUIDE

Provider's Name, Specialty: **Date: (put in upper right corner)**

PART 1: Reason for your office visit today: List all the symptoms. (ex: fever, pain, headache)

Chief Complaint (CC): Pain in low back

O – started 3 days ago when I leaned over to pick something up
L – in low back
D – constant pain
C – burning and aching, not sharp
A – walking makes it worse
R – tried ibuprofen without relief, R (radiation) – none
T – had this same thing 5 years ago due to a work injury
S – now the pain is causing nausea and I have tingling in both legs

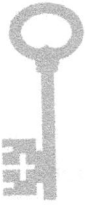

Do not wait until your appointment to fill out your OLD CARTS. When you have a *chief complaint*, grab a sheet of paper and put it on the refrigerator with the complaint name and date. Then if it gets better, just throw it in your medical folder drawer. If it doesn't, take it with you to tell your provider exactly when it started.

This method is so simple and saves so much time, it is a shame that more patients will not do this for their doctors.

HINT: Providers cannot stand it when a patient does not know how long their complaint has been going on. For example, if you have been short of breath for one hour versus one year is a major difference in how your treatment will go. You must know the exact time within two or three days of when the symptom started. Never tell your provider "a while." This has no meaning and here's why:

A patient comes in with a cough. It's been going on for "a while." When the provider asks exactly how long, the patients says, "Two weeks." The next patient comes in with a headache. She, too, says it's been going on for "a while." The physician asks exactly how long the headache has been going on and the patient says, "Six months." So, you see, providers hear this all day long and that one phrase, "a while," means nothing to the provider because it means so many different things to different people.

Step 4. Packing Your Medical Office Bag

Here is the list of seven things you should bring to your provider's office:

→ A good book to read

→ Warm clothes (because the office and exam room are cold). Layer your clothes so you can add more or take off some as needed.

The nurse told me to take off my shoes and step up on the scale. I said I needed something to cover the scales, as I was not putting my bare feet on it. I told her that otherwise I would keep my shoes on. She scowled and got several paper towels to cover the scale. Do not step on that scale barefoot. Wear socks on your feet, because when you get weighed in, your feet get contaminated. It makes me shudder to see how much fungus and bacteria step on the scale in a doctor's office every day.

(And another point: Do not walk through airport security without socks on. If you could see the fungal infections in toes and feet, you would consider socks, shoes, and TSA-precheck from now on.)

→ Your paper or Office Visit Guide form from the Patient Best® Medical History Book showing your chief complaint and all others

→ A list of all your medicines. We will talk more about this later.

→ Insurance cards and driver's license and your checkbook or credit card or cash for the co-pay

→ A snack (especially if you are diabetic and will need to eat)

→ A bottle of water

Okay, we are ready!! Now let's learn the seven steps of every healthcare provider's office visit, whether specialist, dentist, primary doctor, or even physical therapy. These steps are the same across all provider professions. Why? Because insurance will not pay unless all these steps are accounted for in your chart.

Arrival time!

The Seven Steps of Every Office Visit

Step 1. The Receptionist

You walk up to the front desk. This receptionist has a hundred things to do at once. The best you can do is sign in and wait to be called. Be patient if he or she is on the phone. Someone is calling in for something and the receptionist must take a message or look up a piece of information. If you sign in and sit down, the front desk personnel will call you if they need anything.

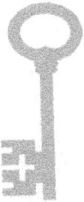

When the receptionist does check you in, you will be asked, "Has anything (on your chart) changed since you were here last?" You are *not* to answer that question! Because you do not know the answer! Do you really know what they are referring to? Did they show you their computer? No. Therefore, you are going to say, "I don't know. What are you referring to?"

A proactive patient went in to her doctor's office and the receptionist asked this very question. The patient turned to the receptionist and said, "Yes, as a matter of fact, quite a bit has changed. I changed the color and style of my hair, and I got new glasses. My husband and I moved into a nice condo last month, and my oldest grandchild graduated from college."

Because you do not know what is in the receptionist's computer, you cannot answer this question. This is where mistakes are made. Over 70 percent of one emergency room's charts had wrong telephone numbers, so that they could not reach patients to tell them to come back in for whatever reason.[1] The front desk is supposed to specifically read out the information and confirm its content, but they always seem to ask, "Has anything changed?" Do not answer yes or no. Ask them what they are referring to.

I saw one receptionist slam a paper on the counter with the patient's name and telephone number and ask him to review and sign it. She was not about to go over the information verbally. This may be a more accurate way of making sure the information is correct. I'm not so sure that slamming it on the counter was necessary.

Once you have signed in, look around the waiting room and see who is there. Note who came in behind you.

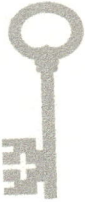

I watch patients sit for hours without noticing that patients are coming in behind them and being taken back while the earlier patient is still waiting. Some practices have multiple providers and some providers work faster than others, so it truly depends on whom you are going to see. Having said this, it is always a good idea to check back with the receptionist if you are still waiting and everyone has now gone home. This happens a lot. The staff does not mean to skip you, but it happens.

Step 2. Being Taken Back to the Exam Room

First, ask the person's name and position if the person does not introduce him- or herself. It is always nice if this person does so.

The person may take you to the exam room or may ask you to step on the scale and get weighed. Here's the rub: Why do you need to get weighed?

Many patients hate the office scale. Most tell their providers that the scale is wrong and they do not weigh so much. Providers do not care. While they know the scale is slightly wrong, it is not enough to make a difference. They are weighing you for two reasons. The first is so they can get one of many vital signs to show the insurance company that they checked all the boxes, so that they can get paid. Yes, this is one of the 178 mandates your insurance company expects of your provider. More important is the second reason for which your provider looks at your weight: to see if it has significantly changed since your last "wrong-weight" weigh-in. Your doctor may then tell you either to lose or to gain weight, to exercise more and drink more water.

> One patient went to the ophthalmologist and got weighed in. The ophthalmologist came in after forty-five minutes, told the patient to look up, then look down, and then said the patient's eyes were good and left. When patient requested a copy of his office visit, he was shocked to see that the ophthalmologist had noted that he had spent time talking to the patient about his weight. This was not the case but was now designated on his chart.

Next the back-office person will take your other vital signs. This may include your pulse, temperature, respirations, blood pressure, and/or pain rating on a scale of 1 to 10. Your provider needs this information to confirm that you are stable and in good condition but also so the boxes can be checked for the insurance company.

Once you are in the room, you are asked to sit on the exam table. If the back-office person is allowed, they will go over your medications, ask if you are pregnant (yes, this is true for boys and girls), and go over the following parts of your chart.

Medications: Most back-office personal cannot take this information out of your chart when you discontinue a medication. Usually only the doctor or provider can do this, so ask if this is the case. Major medical errors are caused because medication lists are wrong.

Chief complaint: "What brings you in today?" HINT: Do not say, "My wife." We know someone told you to come in and get checked out, but we want to know your chief complaint. This is also called the HPI (history of present illness).

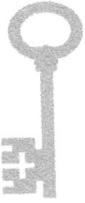

Get out your paper that you brought with you. It should have your OLD CARTS already written down for your office visit. Look over the OLD CARTS. Start reading this to the back-office person. Keep this paper out, because you are going to need it again.

Family, surgeries, hospitalizations, social history — the back-office person wants to know this and update your chart.

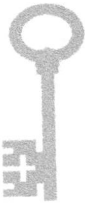

Do *not* just say yes and no, but ask this person what is in their chart and correlate it with what is in your own medical history records.

Repeatedly, a provider will find mistakes and incomplete histories on the patient. Remember, your doctor does not know that you went to the cardiologist, who changed your medication; that you went to the ER for a heart attack; or that you had a knee replacement since last seeing her for a quick checkup. All this information must go into your chart. Even after the back-office person has asked you all this, little will get into your chart. Ask this person to review it with you and to show you your records on the computer screen.

If more back-office personnel would slow down and put information in accurately, charts would not kill so many people. It is not the fault of this person, nor of the provider. Again, healthcare now dictates how fast patients need to be moved like cattle through the office visit. The office personnel not only have to escort you to an exam room but need to move to the next patient and let the doctor know you are ready. They are on to the next patient and trying to keep one step ahead of their doctor. Remember, the doctor has to move fast, too.

Your healthcare office is also timing you. The front desk must put in the time you checked in. The back-office person must enter the time you were brought to the back. The doctor must enter the time he or she entered the exam room, and finally, the time you checked out and received your walking papers. The healthcare big-business employer wants to monitor how fast the staff can keep moving cattle, I mean patients, through the line.

Did you know that patients fall off the table? So why does the back-office person consistently tell the patient, "The doctor will be right in" and then leave? Never has worse nonsense been spoken! When the doctor or provider does finally get to the exam room, guess where the patient is. On the floor? Close. Yep! In the chair. Why? Because the patient is mad and tired of waiting on an uncomfortable exam table for the doctor.

In truth, it will take the doctor about another forty-five minutes, on average, to get to you once you have been roomed. Now you know why you brought a snack, a good book, and a bottle of water.

As I, in my role as provider, was passing a nurse in the hall, she was coming out of an exam room with the magic words "The doctor will be right in." So I stopped her and told her to go back in and ask the patient to move to a chair, where he would be more comfortable, and offer some water and a blanket if he was cold. She looked at me like I was nuts. I then explained to her that I still had to go read an x-ray and discharge one patient, I had another patient I was waiting on lab work for, and I hadn't gotten to the third patient, who had multiple chronic diseases, so it would be at least forty-five minutes before I would be able to see the patient she had just left. You should know doctors run late and it's because there are more tests, conversations, and complaints thrown into each and every patient visit.

Let's fix this. . . .

You as the patient have now gotten through steps 1 and 2 with flying colors. You checked in correctly. You got through the call-back step with your chart in hand and your notes and OLD CARTS.

Now the doctor or midlevel enters the room. After introductions, the provider will wash her or his hands and log in to the computer.

The next four steps are completed by your doctor or provider. You really do not have to do anything, just understand what they are doing and why it is important.

This part of the office visit is recorded with a SOAP note. It consists of step 3 through 6:

Step 3 — **S**ubjective; Step 4 — **O**bjective; Step 5 — **A**ssessment; Step 6 — **P**lan. Let's review these next steps.

Step 3. Subjective

Your doctor will ask you the same set of questions the back-office person asked, but more important, the doctor will stop your conversation to clarify, listen, and listen again. With your OLD CARTS still in hand, tell your provider exactly what your complaint is. What your doctor is trying to do is discern why you are there, what is causing the problem, and whether it might be dangerous for you.

After you have gone through your OLD CARTS (again), the doctor will ask you questions and look at your chart to see your problems and your other illness. He or she will also look at your medications. All of this is in an effort to figure out whether any of these medications, illnesses, or social habits could be causing your problems.

Let's take an example. Let's say you go to the office for a cough you've had for two months. You doctor wants to see whether you smoke (*social*), whether you have ever had pneumonia or other lung diseases (*chronic medical problems*), and whether you take medications like an over-the-counter antihistamine for allergies (*medications*). All this has to be known to your provider. Then the concerns start. Could this be just a cough, pneumonia, lung cancer, heart issues, or allergies? Each one of these items has to correlate with what you tell your doctor.

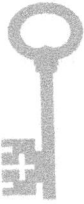

Now you can see why your chart is so important. Make sure the back-office person has changed the appropriate items to reflect your accurate health. Suppose your doctor wants to do a chest x-ray? Do you have a copy of an old one you can show him, so he can compare the two? Doctors like to compare records to see if there are any changes. We will talk more about this later.

I once had a patient come in with chest pain. His EKG that day was abnormal. By the way, many EKGs show variances; normal EKGs are found in textbooks for teaching purposes only. Anyway, this patient was getting ready for a trip to the emergency room and a $7,000 bill to boot. But then he did something I never had seen before. He reached into his wallet and pulled out a copy of his last EKG from his cardiologist's office. He explained to me that his cardiologist said to always keep this with him, as this prevented him from getting ordered to the emergency room. And he was correct. Because the two EKGs were identical even though abnormal, they were not the cause of his visit, his heart could be ruled out as the problem, and he was not sent to the ER.

Step 4. Objective

This means exam time. Now your physician or provider is going to examine those parts of your body which you are complaining about. They will also be watching how you move from the chair to the exam table. They will be looking at your skin, how you turn your head, your ankles, and your hands and feet. Physicians are very observant. Within seconds of entering an exam room, most providers have identified any "alarms" they have to address.

Several things you want to do during this six-minute visit. When the physician is listening to your heart and lungs, do NOT speak. Why? Because your provider cannot hear you. Your words are garbled and sound like a bad fast food speaker through a stethoscope. When a physician needs to listen to your neck, NEVER speak. You will deafen the examiner, as your vocal cords are there.

When you lie down, put your hands to the side. The examiner needs to look, hear, and feel your belly.

When the physician is done examining you, ask what she or he found.

For example, if the doctor looks in your ears, ask whether you have wax in them.

Part of Step 4 (Objective) is also your labs and imaging studies such as x-rays, CT scans, and MRIs. Your examiner will look over all your reports to determine if they show anything disturbing or abnormal and discuss them with you.

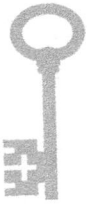

Know that your physician knows what is best for you and can discern what needs to be discussed and what does not. If you do not understand something, it is certainly okay to ask your provider to explain the results to you. Do not assume "normal" means normal. Ask your providers to look at the report and see if there is anything worrisome about the labs, x-rays, or any other reports you might have. You need a professional set of eyes to look at your report and give you a layman's explanation for what is on that report.

The easiest items for you to become familiar with are your blood pressure readings, your A1c (if you are diabetic) and your weight. You should know these at every office visit. Be sure to write them down on the back of the OLDCARTS paper you carry.

Step 5. Assessment
This means diagnosis. The physician will need to give you a diagnosis, or assessment, in order to complete your chart and get reimbursed by the insurance company. In fact, many electronic medical records require the provider to include a diagnosis with every medication they prescribe for you.

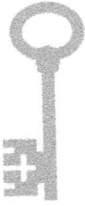

Always ask the provider what diagnoses you have been given. Also ask which diagnosis is new and which are old diagnoses that were already in your chart. Many charts show a wrong diagnosis because the patient does not keep track of this. A real problem arises when the insurance company raises your premiums and you do not understand why. Take at a look at the diagnoses they read in your medical records. Your chart may very well be the culprit.

Also, understand that in 2015 the government came out with a whole new set of ICD codes for billing purposes (International Class of Disease — 10th Revision). We will discuss this in depth in chapter 10. You will then learn why this is so important.

Many patients are shocked when I show them the computer and they look at all the diseases they have in their chart. The list can easily have thirty items even though the patient may have only six diseases or disorders. For example, one doctor put in "obesity," while another doctor put in "obesity due to excess calories," while another doctor put in "obesity without chronic disease," while another doctor put in "obesity with BMI 30 – 34.5," and another doctor put in "obesity with comorbidities." There are thousands of ICD codes and every provider uses her or his favorites. But when they do so, you chart ends up with multiple diagnoses for the same problem, depending on the number of different doctors you see. I have seen multiple patients ask me to please remove a wrong diagnosis from their chart. To get this off the chart and out of the insurance records is a gargantuan task and takes time and connections with the right people. How hard is this? The problem parallels identity theft and cleaning up your medical records is just as hard as cleaning up your identity. Many patients now hire a patient advocate who specializes in medical charting just to be sure charts are always monitored and correct. The disconnect between diagnoses in your medical chart and problems you really have is part of the miscommunication and charting errors we discussed in earlier chapters. Bad charts can and will kill you.

Step 6. Plan

The plan is what the physician and providers will tell you to do. Sometimes it's as simple as "Check back with me in a few weeks," and sometimes it's a referral to a specialist, a medication, physical therapy, labs, imaging studies, and so on. There are a multitude of plans your physicians can order.

Each plan should have a diagnosis. Why is the doctor ordering this? Is it necessary?

We will dedicate all of chapter 9 to doctors' orders, because orders can devastate you mentally, physically, or emotionally. The right orders can save your life.

For now, just keep track and write down what the doctor or provider is asking you to do. Make sure all your questions are answered.

Step 7. Check-out Time!

Either the provider or the back-office personnel will walk you out to the front desk. You last step in the process is *always* to stop at the front desk. Ask for a copy of "today's office visit" to be sent to your home. Do not ask for a copy of your chart. That's a massive amount of information and you have your own chart already. You need only today's visit record, one part of your whole chart.

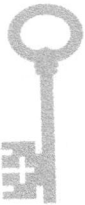

Many receptionists will tell you that your visit is online and you can find it there. This is not necessarily true. What your doctor charts about you and what you read online can be two different things. Your own chart must stay up-to-date and this means you must have the record of today's office visit.

This record should be mailed to you within the week. Your provider may not have time to finish completing the record of your visit until the end of that day or the next. If you do not get a copy within the week, check back with the office. Always get the name of the receptionist you spoke to so that if you need to call back, you can talk directly to that same person.

Also, in order to know you have the correct paper, you must see the physical exam (*Objective*) on it. If you do not see this, then you have an incomplete visit or record. This is useless, as all providers need to see steps 3 through 6, the SOAP note, in your own personal medical chart for it to be considered complete

We will also speak to the cost of the plans or orders your doctor is requesting of you, in chapter 9.

CHAPTER 6

Your Medications and How the Pharmacy Works

"**A**sk your doctor . . ." "Tell Your doctor . . ." Unless you do not own a television, you have seen the advertisements for drugs on television. Some call them medications. Why do manufacturers advertise on television? Because it works. What doesn't work is the price of the drug. Many times, patient unknowingly ask doctors about a drug they have seen on television and find the price is so exorbitant they can't afford it anyway.

What is especially interesting about medications are the side effects they have. All have side effects. By law, advertisements must state the side effects of these drugs. In these ads, side effects are always listed while the person is laughing, running, eating, or enjoying friends and family. I love how they say, "May cause nausea, vomiting, or diarrhea" while the actors are enjoying a picnic in a park, as far from a restroom as one can get. The power of visual is much stronger than the power of audio.

Because of the variables in human bodies, habits, and food intake, it is impossible to know how these chemicals will act within one system or the next. My dad always waited six months before prescribing a new drug. He said it was a good way to see what the true side effects were, once it was taken by millions of people.

This country would do well to get drug ads off television, but this is not going to happen. According to Dr. Rich Parker, this is a matter of free speech and companies have a right to advertise.[1] Pharmaceutical companies spend $5 billion a year advertising to the consumer and another 45 billion advertising to medical providers. Cigarette ads were removed in 1970, and hopefully they will not return to television. Big-business healthcare and television are all about the money. Television is not about to lose its revenue from pharmaceutical companies. So the advertisements stay.

The good news is that you can do something to protect yourself. Your pharmacist or specialized patient advocate can do a medication reconciliation for you. Medication reconciliation means the pharmacist or patient advocate will look at all medications you take and for what diagnoses, then compare side effects, check for drug interactions. and review cost savings. Medicare and most private-pay insurance companies will pay for the pharmacist to do this. Find out how often you can get this medication counseling. To avoid safety concerns, it is recommended that you have this done after every discharge from the hospital and every time one of your providers changes your medications. Do not forget to include all your over-the-counter medications as well. They have side-effects, too. Remember the commercials on television for over-the-counter medication? Next time watch, and you will hear the side effects of these medications, too. If you are at the pharmacy and cannot remember which over-the-counter medications you take, then grab a basket, go aisle by aisle, and grab one of each of your medications, place it in the basket, and let the pharmacist add these to your list.

Many patients have read news articles that say doctors are influenced by pharmaceutical companies and pharmacists, and some even get kickbacks when they prescribe their drugs. Most physicians do not practice this way. In 2008, a movement to ban pharmaceutical companies from giving pens and trinkets to physicians ended an era of influence on physicians. This movement began among physicians who felt this was not in the best interest of their practices and patients. Congress might serve their constituents better if they, too, took notice and banned lobbyists from exerting such influence. It is important to know that the only influence most physicians encounter now is from free drug samples and food for their staff at lunch.

Now let's talk about the right pharmacy and pharmacist you need in order to stay away from medication errors.

Most drugs have side effects and may have interactions with other drugs. It is imperative that you have a local pharmacist you can trust to watch your back when it comes to medications. If you are using more than one pharmacy, you increase your risk of experiencing a medical error or mistake.

For example, let's say you use a mail-order company for long-term medications, a local pharmacy for short-term medications, and then from time to time you go to the corner urgent care when you can't get into your healthcare system. So you are now using three pharmacies. These pharmacies do not talk to one another. Therefore, you do not know what the drug interactions may be. If you are continuing to take all the medications prescribed by them and then adding over-the-counter drugs on top of these, you will surely have some interactions. A rule of thumb is "More than ten medications equals a serious interaction." This includes all over-the-counter medications, too.

So let's talk about the pharmacist, an important part of your medical care. These are highly skilled men and women who have spent years studying their profession. It is extremely hard to get into pharmacy school. A pharmacist must be licensed in his or her state. Pharmacists must be board certified. Not only do they go to undergraduate college for four years, but then they have to complete five years of pharmacy graduate school. They have a doctoral degree in pharmaceutical studies. They have studied biochemistry with clinical applications. They partner with doctors and suggest which medications will and won't work for a patient and why. They work closely with clinical studies for safety and efficacy. They are found every day in retail stores across America, as well as hospitals, clinics, and pharmaceutical companies, where they support your physician and you.

Please do not yell at the pharmacist about the cost of your medication. There is a major misconception that pharmacists set the price of your prescriptions. Nothing could be further than the truth. Pharmaceutical pricing is complex, opaque, and insane. It is very hard on most pharmacists when a patient yells at them, because they know that when they tell a patient the prescription costs $700, the patient isn't going to be able to pay that. And yet they have no alternative. The prices are set by corporate executives who negotiate costs with pharmaceutical companies then add profit to support their pharmacy chains across America.

Here is a short version of how pharmaceutical pricing works. It is not pretty. Pharmacies purchase medications from pharmaceutical companies and then raise prices for the consumer at astronomical levels. Executives called benefit pharmacy managers then negotiate these insane prices for insurance companies and bring the prices back down 70 to 90 percent. So the price is not set at the local level. Nor is it — even more importantly — going to be the doctor who sets the prices. Most physicians, nurse practitioners, and physician assistants do not know the cost of medications or your insurance plan and hardly know what pharmacy you are using. There's no way to know all drug prices and insurance plans. Also remember that these negotiator executives had to negotiate the cost of reimbursement with your insurance company. If your insurance company says that it is willing to pay only as little as possible — let's say $25 for your medicine — then your pharmacy will charge you appropriately. But if your pharmacy has negotiating power and says, "No, we want $300 for that drug," sometimes insurance companies have to buckle and pay that amount. Other times, the pharmacy will need to charge a higher price in order to keep its doors open. It's all give-and-take at the table in someone's boardroom.

Prices can change daily, too. Because of this, it is always important to check with your insurance company to be sure you are going to the right pharmacy.

An advocate who specializes in medication reconciliations and insurance brokering told me he once saved a couple $600 a month. They were both going to the same pharmacy. By her going across the street to a different pharmacy, she saved $600 every month. It can be as simple as that, but most patients do not know to ask. Make sure you are going to the right pharmacy to get your medications.

Another example is cash-only medications. There are more programs entering the market like GoodRx. This company was started to give cash-paying patients a chance to purchase their medications at a lower cost. Patients are catching on to these new savings. Pharmacists are not allowed by the employer to tell you to pay cash and get it cheaper, so you have to ask.

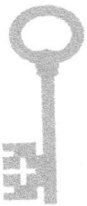

Every time you get a prescription filled, ask the pharmacy if you can get it for less if you do not use your insurance but pay cash. This means you are going to go "off your prescription plan" and explore another cost of the same drug.

Let's say your doctor prescribes a product that is over-the-counter. Now you have three costs of this product. One cost is the cost of the product on the shelf. The second is the cost of the prescribed product under your insurance plan, and the third is the cost of the prescribed product if you offer to pay by cash or credit card (not utilizing your insurance). Try it at different stores and see what the costs are.

GoodRx and many similar companies have websites (e.g., GoodRx. com). Their value is found when you create an account, log in, and compare the prices of your medication to the prices at local pharmacies. You do not need to have an account nor will you be inundated with hundreds of emails. GoodRx is just giving you a choice to pay less for your medications. There are now several other prescription discount coupon plans popping up. You may need to check with every plan to see which is best for you and which is best for each medication you take. Daunting, right?

A patient came in to urgent care. She was distressingly ill with an upper respiratory infection. She was a cash-paying patient with little money to pay for prescriptions. She would already spend $200 out of pocket just to walk through our doors. With a little time on our hands, I walked her through the GoodRx program. We looked up the medications I would be prescribing for her. Here's what the prices were in three local pharmacies:

Pharmacy	Product 1	Product 2	Product 3
X	Free	$79	$110
Y	$30	$49	$7
Z	$89	$9.40	$90

She was kind enough to call me back to say that this program worked, and she received her three products for less than $17 total.

So how do these discount coupon programs work? Basically, insurance companies would rather not pay for your drugs. They offer a discount if you will pay cash and leave them alone. Let's say your drug under the prescription plan costs you $20. Your pharmacy also has to file for reimbursement and paperwork then has to be processed. If you pay cash, the pharmacy may discount the drug to $4. This saves you $16. The insurance company gives the discount coupon program ten cents for the transaction and calls it a day, saving time, paperwork, and salaries. Pharmaceutical companies don't care what you pay for the medication.

They have already set their price with the insurance industry or the discount coupon program.

Pharmacies are now found on every street corner. Gone are the churches, which have moved to the middle of the block as mega churches. Pharmaceutical companies make huge profits and lobby strongly in Washington, DC, to keep their profits in place. Pharmacists' associations also lobby to keep their interests alive. The health insurance industry doles out $157 million in lobbying; these two health entities together spend about $397 million a year in lobbying activities.[2]

> I once had a pharmacist tell me that his grocery store pharmacy made so much money that it paid for the lease of the real estate the grocery store was on, all the employees' salaries, and the heating, cooling, plumbing, and electricity used by the grocery store. The only cost to the grocery store was the food products, and those, of course, were marked up for profit.
>
> All the other products in a drugstore are window dressing to entice you into the store. The pharmacy holds the key to profit.

Similarly to doctors, pharmacists used to know their patients. Now, pharmacists are filling hundreds and sometimes thousands of prescriptions in a twelve-hour shift. Keeping good pharmacists is a challenge for any retailer. Pharmacists, like doctors, are under extreme pressure to work faster and harder and bring home high customer satisfaction scores without the safety net and personal touch they were so used to. Pharmacies in retail stores have high turnover and burn-out due to large corporations' demands for profit. As do doctors, pharmacists have overwhelming student loan debt.

There are financial incentives to push generics, as this saves the customer money and pharmacists get a generic bonus at the end of the year for giving you generics over brand-name medications. One of my friends told me her father, a pharmacist, made $40,000 bonus money at the end of the year from this. He didn't need it, so he doled it out to his pharmacy staff.

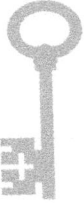

It is critical that you find and engage a pharmacist to be your advocate. Many patient advocates have at least three pharmacists they turn to for help when their clients are changing medication or prescribed new ones. Find a pharmacist you can trust. Give this person a list of all your medications from all your different mail-order and other pharmacies. Include the over-the-counter medications, vitamins, and supplements as well. Do not forget the protein shakes full of vitamins. They may be interfering with the absorption of some of your medications. Ask your pharmacist or your patient advocate to sort this out for you.

Refills

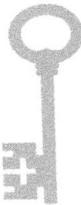

Never leave the pharmacy counter before checking your medication. Open the bottle, look at the pills, and make sure they are the same as what you used to take. Take a picture of each of your different pills and the bottle it comes in, so you can compare every refill with the last one.

Your doctor and you decide whether the medications you are taking have real benefit. Take, for example, your blood pressure medicine. It is finally doing the job and lowering your blood pressure. You get your prescription filled and find that this new pill is different in color, size, and shape. You call the pharmacist over to your counter. Why is it different? Most likely, the pharmacy chain is dealing with a new generic manufacturer. The pharmacist tells you it is the same and you can take it. This may be the case, but what about the inactive ingredients such as in the coating any preservatives?

Will the pharmacy take the product back if it no longer works or has new side effects? Probably not. Will the generic company take the product back? Yes. Most pharmaceutical companies take products back and give credit back to the pharmacy. Why pharmacies do not pass this refund policy on to the consumer is not clear. Ask the pharmacist to give you the name and number of the pharmaceutical company in case you need to return the product. Many of these drugs are manufactured in other countries, so your chances of getting reimbursed are slim but there is hope. Every pharmacy works with a middle man called the pharmacy benefits manager, who works for the drug and medical supply warehouse. These are regionally located. Ask the pharmacist who is the supplier of your products and see if you can get a refund through the supplier.

Formulary

Whether working with a hospital or a pharmacy, insurance companies work from a list of drugs that are preapproved and they are willing to pay for. This list is called the formulary. These medications tend to be in three price tiers.

→ Tier 1: Generics, the cheapest

→ Tier 2: Brand-name, more expensive

→ Tier 3: Most expensive and most likely either a new drug or advertised on television

Bring a copy of your formulary with you to your doctor's office. These men and women are the *only* professionals who can prescribe medications, so be prepared with your list of what they can order and not order.

I walked into an exam room and the patient was standing there waiting for me. On the exam table, the counter, and even covering the sink were one-sheet papers all laid out for viewing. I asked her what all this was. She explained that these were her formularies from her insurance company. If I was going to prescribe any medications she wanted to be sure they were from *tier 1*, her least expensive choice.

Within minutes we had her list reviewed and her prescriptions ready. She knew her preparedness was saving her time and money.

SHORT-TERM VERSUS LONG-TERM MEDICATIONS

Many patients today are living longer than ever before. Surprisingly, most are not taking medications. They walk daily, socialize daily, and drink plenty of water for good hydration. Unfortunately, there are those patients who need medications. No matter what they eat or how much they exercise, they cannot control their disease or disorder without medications. They spend large sums of money every month for their prescriptions.

These are typically known as long-term medications and they are taken over thirty days. Most are taken month after month for years. The conditions they are used to control are known as "chronic" diseases.

It is important to separate out medications you are taking for chronic diseases from the "short-term" medications such as antibiotics, creams for a rash, over-the-counter pain medications, and symptom-relief medications for colds, cough, and flu — i.e., medications you are taking for short-term (acute) disease. Here's an example showing why:

The patient returns to her primary care office every year with the same urinary tract infection. Her doctor notes that she has been on the same short-term antibiotic medication multiple times. She then tells him that she also goes to an urgent care facility for the same problem. When she can't get an appointment with him, she just goes there.

Her bacteriuria (bacteria in urine) may be resistant to her antibiotics and she may need a new product. Without knowing what she is taking, it is hard for the doctor to know what to try next. The added conundrum is that, if she is building resistance to antibiotics, this may land her in the hospital on IV antibiotic treatment every time she gets an infection, unless she keeps a medical record of her antibiotic usage.

It is also a good idea to keep track of medications used, to know which ones worked and which didn't. Some patients think of a drug's failure to work as an "allergy," but this is not correct. Over 90 percent of patients who say they are allergic to PCN (penicillin) are not. They were allergic to the preservative when they were little. Perhaps the preservative is now removed and newer drugs no longer have it.

The best way to find out what you are allergic to is to see your allergist; ask your primary care doctor for this advice and referral. Remember, too, allergy testing is only as good as the day you have the test. What this means is that anyone at anytime can develop a true allergy. You can walk out of an allergist's office and not be allergic to bee stings and the next day swell up like a birthday balloon when stung.

The important idea behind allergy testing is to know what you are truly allergic to and what is truly just intolerance.

Also, if you do get allergy testing, ask about preservatives and who tests for those. New companies are doing multiple sensitivity testing for better chronic disease control. See www.reversemydiabetes.net to learn more about how Denise Pancyrz controls sugar elevations by keeping sensitivities in check.

Intolerance is a side effect of a drug. It can be any of the following and more:

Nausea

Vomiting

Diarrhea

Muscle Weakness

Cough

Allergy

Upset Stomach

Cost

Medication Interaction

Headaches

Rash

Bloating

This list is endless.

Over-the-Counter Medications

Many patients forget to address the over-the-counter vitamins, supplements, and minerals they are taking. Nor do they think to tell their doctors about the pain medications or medications for relief of cough, cold, and flu-like symptoms they have taken or currently take.

There are multiple reasons a pharmacist or doctor must know about all drugs you ingest. Medications have side effects. Many of the over-the-counter medications were once prescription drugs for good reason. Some were once illegal but are now legal in some states.

The following is a list of reasons for caution: reactivity, absorption, side effects, synergism, and cross-intolerance. To be as safe as possible, all these possibilities must be addressed one at a time for each medication.

Finally, should you have an emergency and need to call 911, the emergency medical technicians (EMTs) must know what medications you are taking. If you put your pills in a pill-sorting container, they have no idea what your pills are. Please always keep your pill bottles available. It is highly recommended that you get a large zip-lock bag, label it "Medicines," and put all your pill bottles in it, even after you empty them. This way, if you have to go to the emergency room, you can take the bag with you, even if the pills are still sitting at home in your pill-sorting container.

CHAPTER 7

Hospitalizations, Urgent Care, and Emergency Room Visits

Hospitalizations

Hospitalizations are extremely dangerous to the patient, yet a necessary evil. When you are hospitalized, you must have a family member or professional patient advocate to secure your safe return to your home. Understand that hospitals do not want you in their facility for any longer than your insurance will pay for. The number of days is often based on your diagnosis. This means that the hospitalist is focused on your discharge. The biggest question is, "What will it take to get this patient well and out of the hospital?" While this is a great question because you do not want to be in the hospital any longer than necessary, the problem is the discharge.

Know that hospitals have a thirty-day "Readmission Penalty" they suffer if you return to the hospital within thirty days of discharge. They will not get paid by insurance if this occurs. They have got to secure a living place for you that will not give you the chance to "bounce back," as it is called in the hospital administration profession.

A young man goes in to the hospital with lower back pain. He is complaining that his legs are tingling and numb. The doctors cannot figure out what is wrong with this young healthy man. They keep him comfortable with pain medication for three days before they finally call in a specialist who recognizes the paralyzing disorder called *cauda equina*. By this time it is too late, and the young man is in a wheelchair the rest of his life.

This brings up another point that must be addressed at this time. When a physician does not know what is wrong with the patient, it is time to find someone who does. Is a misdiagnosis worse than no diagnosis? It depends. Every case is different. A better question would be, "*Is* what doctors are doing working? Or is it just masking the symptoms with medications and procedures?" All patient advocates know that if the doctor cannot find the answers, then a specialist has to be called in. Time is of the essence.

Many physicians rely on patient advocates to help them through the hospitalization of a loved one. Story after story emerges of physicians telling the hospitalist that they are concerned about their loved one and being ignored. One physician told me he had to call in a professional patient advocate to get the treatment his loved one needed, because the hospital staff continued to ignore his concerns even though he was a physician.

Hospitalists are overworked and charting takes up over a third of their time. They have a high rate of turnover, simply because the top-heavy hospital administrators are constantly changing policies based on hospital ratings and not on good medical practice. One hospitalist told me he had to see close to twenty patients in one shift. This includes addressing all the labs, imaging studies, and other work-ups for each critically ill patient.

A major disadvantage of hospitalizations is infection rates. Some of the best-known hospitals in this country have the worse infection rates. There are now professional patient advocates who serve patients by looking for the safest hospital and specialist to get needed procedures done.

A physician had uncontrolled diabetes and sought relief from constant excruciating pain in his legs. He was told that the only way to end the pain was to amputate both legs and then get prosthetics to replace them. He told a patient advocate to whom he refers a lot of his patients about this. The advocate was shocked that he had accepted this treatment plan and was ready to move forward with it. She immediately located the best microvascular surgeon in the country, and this doctor restored the man's legs to full vascular supply. Microsurgery is a highly specialized practice. This surgeon spent an extra two years perfecting this surgery and is nationally known for his expertise.

Finding an advocate who can offer you choices and knows the connections to get you where you need to be is good medicine. When insurance companies want to deny a surgery or hospitalization, then it is time to find a patient advocate who specializes in turning insurance denials into approvals. Insurance companies have ratings just like hospitals and doctors. In today's social media, insurance companies want to maintain a good image as much as the next guy.

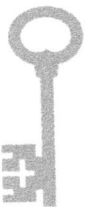

There is no Christmas in July in medicine. July is the deadliest time to get sick. Medical students have just graduated and are now practicing physicians in their residencies. While they have supervision, they are on their own. They are treating you and still rather new at their profession. Some are overworked. Their tired endurance allows them to see patient after patient without breaks. Whether they graduated at the top of their class or at the bottom, it is not your decision whom you will be seeing. Yes, some of them do know what they are doing, but the majority order labs and more labs because they don't know much else to do. They don't have the experience yet, so just be forewarned: I've known doctors and directors to actually go on vacation in July because, as one doctor literally said, "I can't stop the residents from killing the patients. So I have earned the right to go on vacation in July. I do it so my staff can handle the residents."

In July, keep an advocate and a second, well-known, experienced doctor by your side.

Emergency Departments and Urgent (Convenient) Care Centers

Patients are often shocked at the expense incurred with an emergency room visit. Worse yet is the cost of the ambulance ride to get there. In Kentucky, at the time of this writing, ambulance services cannot charge the patient. It is law that when a service receives tax dollars to operate, then it cannot charge the recipient for its services. Police and fire departments are paid with taxes and do not charge individuals for their services, so should ambulance services that accept tax dollars also charge patients?

Patients should be aware of whether their insurance will or will not pay for ambulance service. Also understand that in some states, ambulances will not take you to the emergency room of your choice but may take you to the one with the shortest wait time. It depends on your urgency and need for medical attention.

Because some emergency rooms make emergency medical personnel wait along with other patients if it is not a true emergency, the ambulance personnel may decide whether you are a "true" emergency and, if not, encourage you to drive yourself so they will not have to wait with you in the emergency waiting room.

Many people believe that if they call an ambulance, they will get into the emergency room faster. This is no longer the case. Emergency departments take the most emergent cases first. Patients and ambulances will wait their turn. People often ask urgent care doctors, "Will I have to wait?" It always depends on how severe the situation is.

Urgent care or convenient care centers are becoming more and more prevalent. Due to the overcrowding of primary care offices, more patients seek urgent care for same-day medical treatment. As mentioned earlier in this book, patients will tell their urgent care provider that they tried to get in to their "doctor's office" but were told they might have to wait three weeks. Thus, they use urgent care for convenience. The doctor's office is now called the "healthcare" office; remember, there is no "convenience" in healthcare.

Let's talk about the expense of emergency departments. Patients will say they had to go there because it was after hours or they had nowhere else to go and they needed urgent treatment. The cost adds up quickly. Understand that getting a bill for $8,000 and then being told you have a sprained shoulder is normal. Both bill and pain seem to indicate more than a sprained shoulder. So why is the bill so high? Emergency room physicians and midlevels are some of the most highly skilled and brightest in the medical field. They are trained to act quickly, and they are thorough. They are constantly looking for anything and everything that could be killing you. The main assumption in the emergency room is that *if* you are there, you may be dying. It is their job to be sure you do not die on their watch. Therefore, all your labs, imaging studies, observations, IVs, and everything else they order are to ensure that you will not die that day.

In the emergency room you will have a complete work-up and will be told your diagnosis. If you do not want a large bill, consider going to a convenient care unless, of course, you cannot breathe or are experiencing stroke symptoms, chest or severe abdominal pain, or any other life-threatening event. Calling 911 will get you the quick evaluation you need. Why healthcare does not offer clinics that offer twenty-four-hour care like emergency rooms do, one will never know. Disease does not work on a time clock.

A patient went into the ER with severe pain in his stomach. When the nurse was interviewing him, she asked if he drank. He said he has a glass of wine from time to time. She wrote "alcoholic" on his chart as part of his history. The work-up was focused on alcoholism, which he never had. The patient lay in bed for days under sedation for "withdrawal." No one could figure out what was wrong with him. His family did not have access to a patient advocate, who could have looked at his hospital records. No one knew he was being treated for the alcoholism misdiagnosis. In fact, he had sepsis; when he woke up, he had no hands or feet. The amputations occurred because of the sepsis.

Patients must always have an advocate in the emergency department. Everyone who touches the patient or gives the patient medication should have their names and procedures recorded either by a family member or an advocate. Every single medication given to the patient is for a diagnosis. An appropriate backup safety system would be for a family member to always ask a nurse who ordered any medication a patient is given, and why.

A man called his wife's patient advocate after she lay on a gurney in the hallway of the emergency department for thirty-six hours. He said she had to use the public bathroom, got cold food, and couldn't sleep because the lights were on twenty-four hours a day and the noise was intolerable. He told her patient advocate they were waiting for a room to be found. The advocate arrived and within the hour the wife had her own room, it was confirmed that she had indeed been admitted and was not "under observation," which makes a huge difference, and a discharge plan was being formulated and would be in place by the end of the day.

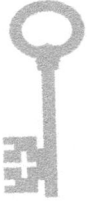

When you are admitted to the hospital, make sure you are actually "admitted" and not "under observation." This relates to your insurance and whether they will pay the bill or not. If you are under observation, your bill is considered to be for out-patient services and is not paid by Medicare Part A but by Medicare Part B. The hospital has to follow guidelines to qualify to admit you versus observe you.

Like Medicare recipients, you have to know your insurance policy and what it will pay for in hospital services versus outpatient services. It makes a huge difference to your wallet. If your hospital can meet the criteria to get you under inpatient admission status, it will do so. Find the admissions officer and do not wait until the bills come in a week or two. Then it may be too late to do anything about the status.

Many patients think they must have been admitted, as they have a private or semi-private room on a wing or upper floor. Do not be fooled by the location of your room. "Admitted" versus "under observation" is a legal distinction made by insurance companies and hospital programs. To be sure whether you or your loved one is actually admitted to the hospital, you must read the paperwork. Many times, as an advocate, I have asked for the paperwork and seen that it indicated "observation," so I got this designation changed and made the change retroactive to the time the patient entered the hospital. Again, insurance does not pay for observation or outpatient services in a hospital at the rate they pay for inpatient services.

CHAPTER 8

Why You Want Your Own Medical Chart

In chapter 4 we discussed the medical chart briefly. Understand that your medical chart holds critical information together for several reasons:

In today's healthcare system, you are a stranger to your doctor. He or she knows you only through your medical chart. If you go to two or more doctors, then they must rely on your chart for accurate information. They must assume the information is accurate because they have no choice. They hope the back-office person got it right. The problem: the information is not accurate.

There is missing information. Electronic medical records do not talk to each other. Many patients assume that if they use a particular medical record system in one office, then everyone who uses that same system also is privy to that information. This is not the case.

Your chart is incomplete. In twelve years of practicing medicine and ten years of advocacy work, I have never seen a complete medical chart. Period. Enough said. You will find gaps and try to retrieve the missing information. Nope, it's gone or destroyed. No one has it anymore. When medical records went online, your paper chart went into the shredder.

Your physician relies on your chart and will diagnose or treat you depending on the conditions found in your chart. Remember that several doctors can list obesity six different ways in your chart. There are over ten thousand ICD diagnosis codes.

There are twenty-two parts to your medical chart. All parts must be checked for accuracy before and after every healthcare visit. This refers to a doctor's visit as well as a visit to or by urgent care, physical therapy, home health, a nurse, a dentist, an ophthalmologist, or other provider. This applies especially to hospitalizations, where all medications are often switched completely, to all new medications. Your chart must be updated to reflect all appointments in healthcare.

Let's go over these twenty-two parts of your medical history. If you have the Patient Best® Medical History Book System (found at www.PatientBest.com), then you already have all twenty-two parts in front of you. Do not give this book to your doctor. It is to be used as your reference guide should your physician need a certain piece of information or want to see a report. Your physician is not interested in reviewing your book and does not have the time.

Part 1. Doctor Visits. Keep track of all of them. Have a copy of your office visit records in chronological order, for easy reference. These visit records should include visits to your specialists, as well.

Part 2. Vital Signs. If you have a blood pressure, which you do, you should keep a copy of those recordings with dates on them. It's also a good idea to keep a record of your weight.

Part 3. Preventive Medical Care. Keep a separate copy of all your preventive medical care. These are healthcare screens like mammograms, bone density, vaccinations, Tuberculosis (TB) tests, pap smears, prostate checks, annual body scans for skin cancer, colonoscopies. Check with your primary care physician or patient advocate for the other screenings you should keep records of here.

Part 4. Short-term Medications. These are medications you have taken for less than thirty days. It is very important that your doctor know which medications you have taken in the past. For example, if you are subject to frequent urinary tract infections, then your doctor needs to know what you last took for one and if that antibiotic truly eradicated the bacteria.

If your child has strep throat often, the pediatrician wants to know the last medication was your child was given so resistance will not develop. Many times, a child ends up in urgent care and the pediatrician does not have access to this chart. So your child's medical chart that you keep gives the pediatrician an all-around view of your child's illnesses and health.

Part 5. Long-term Medications. These are medications taken for over thirty days and should be logged separately from short-term medications. These are for chronic (long-term) disease. What medications currently work for you and what are they taken for?

Part 6. Over-the-Counter Medications. Keep a running list of medications you take from time to time or medications you take only when you want symptomatic relief. These can be pain medications, which may raise blood pressure or cause liver or kidney damage; cough and cold medications, which can raise blood sugar; or allergy medications, which can raise cholesterol. Your doctor runs labs on you to monitor your chronic diseases, and if your next lab is abnormal, then these OTCs may be the cause. If your doctor doesn't know you are taking these medications, he or she may want to do a "complete work-up" on you to find out what is causing the abnormality. This is a waste of time and money and a safety concern if the real cause is just over-the-counter medications.

Benadryl (a Johnson & Johnson product), also known as diphenhydramine, is used for allergies, but one side effect is sleepiness. What the public doesn't know is that diphenhydramine also causes erectile dysfunction.

Johnson & Johnson came out with Tylenol PM® (trademark brand). It contains Tylenol® and diphenhydramine. Its success has been so huge that it and Advil PM® (trademark of Pfizer Consumer Healthcare) are now the biggest selling sleep aids in America. Physicians across the country saw a rise in erectile dysfunction complaints.[1]

Part 7. Allergies. This is a very broad category. Many patients believe they are allergic to medications when they truly are not. It is a dangerous word, "allergy," for the physician to hear. It means a perfectly good medication cannot be used and the physician must entertain a second- or third-choice medication, which may be costlier to you the patient, or worse, not as effective.

Let's look at true allergies. These cause "histamine reactions": rash, hives, itching, difficulty swallowing, shortness of breath, fainting, swelling, or death. This calls for immediate medical attention.

Intolerance refers to a decision not to ingest or apply a medication to your body due to a side effect. This can be one or more of numerous reactions including nausea, vomiting, diarrhea, rash, headache, stomachache, muscle cramps, cross-reaction to other medications you are currently on, heart rate abnormalities, or cost. Sometimes a medication is too expensive until your insurance decides to cover it so that you can afford it. This would be found in the intolerance section of your chart.

Part 8. Chronic Diseases and Past Medical History. This information is critical to your health. In healthcare, physicians often do not know who you are. A specialist knows less about you and your incorrect chart. It used to be that your primary care provider would know you, but six-minute visits do not allow for the time and knowledge the primary care physician needs to get to the root cause of your illness(es). You should know what diseases are in your chart and which are incorrect. So, why does your physician need to know past diseases if you do not have them anymore?

A young woman came in to the urgent care clinic complaining of a dry cough for five days. The doctor examined her and could find no reason for this otherwise healthy woman's cough. She denied congestion, runny nose, allergies, or headache. She was not running a fever. He asked her if she had tried any over-the-counter medications and she said that she had but they did not help. Her lungs were clear, and her respiration was better than normal. As he started to leave, thinking he might just suggest a prescription cough pill, he turned and ask her one more time, "Are you sure you have no lung issues and you have never had anything wrong with your lungs?" It was then that she said, "Oh, yes! I had a pulmonary embolism five years ago and spent a year on blood-thinning medicine." The doctor immediately sent her to the emergency room, where they found two pulmonary emboli (blood clots in the lung), one in each lung. This young woman would have died had she not given this information to her doctor. The doctor told her, "This is the kind of information you lead with when you see all your physicians from now on." Life-threatening events are critical, and every piece of the medical pie has to be known if your physician is going to save your life.

A patient has had cancer. She has now had twenty years in remission when the cancer returns. Her patient advocate is adamant that she get all her medical records. Why? Because her advocate knows that Adriamycin, a cancer treatment drug, cannot exceed a 400-milligram total dose over the lifetime of the patient or it will cause heart failure and eventually kill the patient. When this patient dies, her death certificate will not say, "Medical error due to overdose of

Adriamycin." It will say, "Heart failure." If your physician sees that you have had cancer and now it has returned, you should always be asked about the treatments you had when going through chemotherapy and radiation.

So chronic disease and past and current history lead all physicians to ask about your treatment history. Make sure everything is recorded.

Part 9. Family and Social History. There is no escaping your family when it comes to medicine. Genetics are genetics and you are predisposed to develop what your mom or dad had. Examining this information is called research, and much has been done to ensure that high-risk patients move quickly to begin prevention. One of the biggest mistakes seen is medicine is that this part of your chart is often skipped over.

Also in this section is your social history. This encompasses alcoholism, tobacco abuse, sexual promiscuity, and mental disease. All family members are affected some way. It is important that your medical records show more than what your relatives died from. Your chart should also list any long-standing diseases your family members have suffered from.

There are several big issues surrounding family and social health. Be sure to know what your relatives have gone through physically, mentally, and emotionally. Did they die from medical error or true terminal disease? How could the cause have been prevented?

Family history changes but rarely gets updated in the chart. When was the last time the doctor asked you who in your family died recently and from what?

Social history is just as important and often missed or incorrect. (Remember the twins in chapter 2.) There are several reasons for this and the biggest one is that the patient does not tell the truth or maybe tells just part of it. Lying to your physician can be deadly. In the chapter 2 story, had the patient told her doctor she never smoked when indeed she had, the doctor might have missed the lung cancer that was growing in her chest.

When I went back to school at age fifty to get my PA degree, I used the student health clinic for my annual exams. Every time I went in, the nurse would ask me if I wanted to be tested for sexually transmitted diseases (STDs). Every time, I was shocked they would ask but I always declined. I figured that was protocol for all "students" since this was a college campus. When the third annual visit rolled around and that question came up, I asked the nurse if my theory was correct as to why he asked me about STDs. He said, "Not at all. It says here that you are very promiscuous, have multiple partners and use no protection." I was shocked and dismayed that such mistakes occurred. I requested a copy of my medical office record from then on.

Part 10. Past Surgeries/Hospitalizations. Past surgeries and hospitalizations can involve a large amount of charting. The surgery charting can begin with the patient getting a "preoperative exam" to be cleared for surgery. Then there is the surgeon's note, the anesthesiologist's note, and then postoperative notes by the nurse. Whether the surgery is an emergency, such as open-heart catheterization to put a stent in your heart arteries, or a preplanned surgery like a knee replacement, it is imperative that you get the surgeon's note. If there were any complications, it is important to get all the nursing notes, physical therapy notes, and home health notes following the surgery.

One patient was sure she had had her appendix out and that the pain in her lower belly "could not be appendicitis." Upon evaluation of the surgeon's note, it was discovered that he had left the appendix and taken out only her gallbladder. The surgeon's note will always specify what was taken out; the pathology report will indicate what tissue is being examined, so you know from the pathology report what was sent to the pathologist. Because these reports have so many medical terms, it is important that you have your primary care doctor translate the information to you in terms you can understand.

Another point here is to know that surgeons do not necessarily see you after your surgery. Their main job is to operate. Therefore, you may not see a surgeon again until it is time for your six-week postoperative visit. You may see their midlevel but do not expect the surgeon. Also, your surgeon's number-one concern is always infection, so if you are feeling feverish or have ongoing concerns, tell someone quickly and get evaluated.

Hospitalizations have a huge amount of paperwork. If you are hospitalized, it is best to get your record when you are discharged.

I once had a patient being discharged. As a patient advocate, this is the one time I will definitely walk the patient out of the hospital with family and friends. Usually the patient is in a wheelchair with a nurse pushing the chair. As I always do, we stopped by the medical records office, and we had the patient request a copy of all his medical records. I had no idea where the medical records department was housed in the hospital. Fortunately, the nurse did. She walked us down a deserted hallway and knocked on a twelve-inch by twelve-inch frosted-glass window. There was no sign indicating that this was the medical records office. The window opened and there stood the medical clerk, who asked us what we needed. Both the patient and I were shocked at how this hospital hid this critically important department from its patients.

Hospital records can be more than three inches thick, containing labs, imaging studies, nursing notes, doctor's notes, and surgery notes. They also list all procedures. To simplify these records, you can ask for only the admission record and the discharge summary notes. This will give you the admitting diagnosis and the discharge diagnosis only. If the primary doctor needs more information at a later date, then he or she can request it. But the reason I like to request the complete record is to give it to my client's medical billing advocate so he or she can get a copy of the fees and compare them to what was actually done.

Another important point in hospitalizations to consider is the medications you are given in the hospital. Many times, patients are stabilized and well enough to go home if they continue with the medications they have been given in the hospital. The problem is that when the patient tries to get the prescriptions filled at the corner pharmacy, the cost is so prohibitive that the patient cannot afford them. If you are given prescriptions to be filled upon discharge, call your pharmacy and find out how much they are going to cost you. If you cannot afford them, find your hospitalist and tell him or her that you will need your prescriptions changed to something you can afford. I like to tell the hospitalist that my clients cannot be discharged until they are stabilized and doing well on affordable medications.

Part 11. Emergency Departments and Urgent (Convenient) Care Centers. This the part of your medical record where you will put a copy of your urgent care and emergency room visits. It is best to put them in chronological order and file them with a summary page on the front of this section.

As discussed earlier, imagine that you call your healthcare office (aka doctor's office) for a quick visit and the call center tells you the doctor can see you in three months. Your only choices are the urgent care center or the emergency room.

How do you know whether to go to the emergency room or the urgent care clinic? Well, if in doubt, you can always go to the emergency room, but I'll give you a little heads-up here on what to expect. The New England health institute reported that over 56 percent of emergency room visits were avoidable and patients could have gone to an urgent care center, mini-clinic, or convenient care facility.[2] They are all the same thing. But there is a huge cost difference between the urgent care and the emergency room. The urgent or convenient care runs about $50 to $150 depending on the person's co-pay and level of treatment. But the average emergency room costs vary. In 2013 the average cost was $1200, but that could easily go up to $2100; more often it's around $6000, depending on what the patient has.[3] Also, not only is cost a factor but so is wait time. You will wait in an emergency room anywhere from two to twenty-four hours to be seen. Why? Because if a person comes in with a true emergency — heart attack, inability to breathe, severe abdominal or back pain of some kind, or even loss of consciousness or coma — that person is going to go ahead of you. So you're going to keep getting pushed back and, yes, you can be pushed back twelve or as many as twenty-four hours. It really doesn't matter to the emergency room. They must get the emergencies in first, and if you are sitting there, you are most likely not the emergency. And you need to know that. On the other hand, if you go to an urgent care facility, your wait time may be anywhere from thirty minutes to an hour — not bad.

So what is the decision? Where do I go? Do I go to the emergency room or do I go to urgent care? Costwise, timewise, you go to urgent care. And you go to the emergency room when you have life-threatening injuries or symptoms. What are those and what do they look like? An emergency is when you can't breathe or you have heart or chest or back pain — you must call 911 to get there fast. Remember, if in doubt always call 911 and go by ambulance.

It is very important that your primary care physician know that you are going to the urgent care or the emergency room. Every primary care physician wants you to follow up with him or her once you have finished visiting either the ER or the urgent care clinic. You must bring your discharge papers with you. Better yet, upon discharge, ask that a copy of the provider's visit record be sent to your home. Take the complete visit record, labs included, to your primary care physician. Your physician cannot adequately treat you without knowing what labs and imaging studies or medications were already ordered.

> I worked with a primary care physician in a small community who said it was shameful if his patients went to the emergency room. He expected every midlevel to be on call at all times for his patients so they could avoid going anywhere else. He felt it was an unnecessary burden to place on the emergency department, and if they went there, then they were seriously sick. He also wanted us to keep track of his patients who were admitted and who were sent home.

Another reason you want to keep all your emergency room and urgent care records together in this section is so your primary care physician can look for patterns. Urinary tract infections are very common, and they usually occur are the most inconvenient times. Many patients wait all day thinking, "It will get better." As the sun sets the symptoms only get worse, and then in panic, the patient comes to the urgent care clinic. In fact, after 5 p.m., most of the visits we see in the ER and urgent care are patients who "waited too long" with a urinary tract infection. If you are prone to these infections, it is important that you speak up about this and ask your provider how you can avoid the emergency room or urgent care.

> I once made a patient wait over two hours because she had gone to the emergency room over the weekend and was in our office to follow up with her primary care physician. When we asked her what had happened in the ER, she couldn't tell us. She had no idea what she was treated for. Therefore, we had to call the hospital and get the medical clerk to fax her ER visit record to us. We all waited two hours for it to come.

Part 12. Lab Studies, Cultures, and Pathology Reports. While your medical records may contain years of lab reports, it is really only necessary to keep the most recent three to four labs and then any very abnormal labs, cultures, or pathology reports. There are multiple reasons for keeping your labs. Let's start with the obvious ones first.

The healthcare system is so fragmented that there is no way to keep track of the billions of lab tests that are ordered each year. When you have a blood test ordered, you are often told that if you did not hear back from the doctor's office, then you can assume everything is normal. This is the common error, described earlier, called "neglect." It used to be the norm for a physician to always call you if your lab results weren't normal, and safe medicine was not a concern because the primary care physician could keep track of lab results. Because now the volume of patients and the outsourcing of lab results are dictated by the healthcare administration, it is imperative that all patients have a copy of their results sent to them personally. This is the only foolproof way of guaranteeing that you see the results. While you do not need to know what the results mean, at least the next time you see a doctor, any doctor, you can bring out the lab result and ask the doctor to interpret it. At least you know someone has looked at it.

The second reason you want your lab results kept in one place is for comparison. Physicians like to compare labs, x-rays, MRIs, and many other studies to see if the patient is improving or the condition is worsening or treatment failing.

Another good reason to keep your own set of lab results is to know any diseases you may have had in the past.

One patient had an abnormal pap smear twenty years ago. She kept her results in her medical binder. Her situation cleared up and she had normal pap smears for twenty years. Then one day the results came back abnormal. Knowing what she had in the past made it easy for her doctor to diagnose and treat her as was done before. She did not need a full workup, worry, and added expense. She only needed the same treatment she had twenty years before.

Keep all abnormal lab results in a safe place.

Keeping culture results is very important, too. Treatment is dictated by what you have and what treatment worked previously. For example, you may have a skin infection. The doctor sends it off for a culture. You have a certain bacterium that is resistant to many antibiotics and sensitive to a few. Based on your previous culture report and diagnosis, your doctor may want to order the same medication that worked before.

Part 13. Imaging Studies. This refers to any and all pictures you have had taken of your body. These can be CT scans, MRIs, x-rays, bone density testing, ultrasounds, and so on. The list is endless and includes dental x-rays. These results are mailed to your ordering doctor. You should also get the films. Most of these results can now be given to the patient on a CD. This thought is good until you realize that the physician cannot just stick your CD into a healthcare computer and expect it to work. There are two reasons for this: 1) The computer has too many safety features built into it to protect it from viruses, so no outside hardware is ever opened on a healthcare computer; and 2) The doctor has six minutes to see you and it would take all six minutes and a child to figure out how to open a CD on the computer and get it to work.

Part 14. Extra Medical Services. These are the services you require, such as physical therapy, chiropractic medicine, nonmedical home health, medical home health, transportation, home meals, and the like. Do not forget the name and location of each person who helped you with your medical services, whether the nurse who showed you kindness after your surgery or the physical therapist who knew how to fix your back; these excellent men and women may be hard to find again should you need them. Therefore, it is important that you get and keep their records, too. They have to fill out reports in order to get paid, so request a copy of each report be sent to you, too.

A patient came to her primary care physician complaining of knee pain. The doctor asked her if she had ever had this problem before. She had, indeed, two years before, but it had cleared up with physical therapy. He wanted to know the name of the physical therapist who had helped her. She pulled out her medical history book and had the name and report in seconds. The doctor then asked this patient if this was the person she wanted to go back to. Absolutely she did. So he wrote the order and she was well on her way to recovery.

How many times have we had a great healer in the health field, the doctor who did our shoulder replacement or the nurse who came to the house, but later been unable to remember her name? Get these reports.

Another reason you want these reports is that they tell your current physician if a particular treatment plan worked for you or not. Like imaging studies, these reports can be used to compare how you are doing now with what your bones looked like in the past.

Part 15. Medical Supplies. Why keep information on medical supplies in your chart? What difference does it make? Your medical supplies list tells you, as does your list of medications, what worked in the past and what did not. Whether you keep the item in the closet or not is irrelevant. What is important is that you tried the item and it did not work. If it did work, you would still be using it.

Doctors do not order medical supplies lightly. They know the cost is very high. Insurance companies spend billions of dollars every year to buy these items for you. The medical cost in our last days of life, including the medical supplies we use and medical treatment, is the highest or all our medical care. Hospital beds for the home can cost as much as $400 a day. A CPAP machine for sleep apnea is expensive, as is the test for it.

Write the name and item number of a medical device you have used, or take a picture of it. Keep a record of it in your medical history book. You would be shocked at the newer items coming out that are so well designed and effective, compared to the old ones. Also remember that the fact that you tried a medical supply device and it did not work for you in the past does not mean the newer version won't work for you in the future. Medicine marches on while healthcare fumbles in the wake of progress.

> A patient had a broken ankle. She tried everything to find a knee walker. The insurance would not pay for one. The doctor highly recommended one. They cost $400. She finally found one through an online resale app and bought it secondhand. It worked like a charm.
>
> If you have items in your closet you are no longer using, see about selling them to folks who need them.

Part 16. Eyes. Physicians will tell you that they can keep your heart beating, your lungs breathing, and your colon pooping, but what good is all that if you do not have your eyes to see, your ears to hear, your teeth to chew, and (highlighting your social life) your mind to interact with others.

It is extremely important that these "neck-up check-up" concerns be addressed in your medical book.

It is always a sad day for the American people when big-business medicine puts money before patients. This is the case with the Seniors Have Eyes, Ears, and Teeth Act. This bill, HR3308, was introduced into the House of Representatives in July 2015. Its purpose was to expand Medicare to cover eyeglasses, hearing aids, and dental care. The bill died in the House, as our representatives did not feel this was important enough to put before committee and vote on. Therefore, most folks have to pay out of pocket for their eye exams, glasses, hearing aids, and hearing tests, and dental care is extremely expensive. Then HR 5396 was introduced in 2017, with the same purpose. This bill was also given no chance to pass in the House and move on to the Senate. Congress has looked at the cost of Medicare in terms of how to cut the expense of such a program and pass any costs on to the patient.

Macular degeneration is the most frequent cause of blindness in older adults. There is medical treatment that can slow the process down. It is imperative that you keep a record of your eyesight and how it is progressing throughout your years.

One patient was diagnosed with macular degeneration. She kept all her medical records in her Patient Best⊠ Medical History Book. When she decided to move across the country, she visited her ophthalmologist to get her eyes checked one last time before the move. At the end of the office visit, she requested a copy of her office visit record. When it came in the mail she put it in her medical book. Six months later she moved to California and it came time to establish care with a new ophthalmologist. She took her medical binder with her. The doctor examined her eyes and told her he would see her back in six months to see how her eyes were doing then. She asked him how her eyes were progressing, and he said, "I have no way of knowing, since I do not have your previous medical records." At this point she pulled out her book and gave him a copy of her eye exam records from her most recent visit. After studying them, he looked up and said, "Your eyes have become significantly worse in the last six months. I am starting you on medication immediately to save your eyesight." This woman never did completely loose her eyesight before she passed at ninety-eight.

Understand that while you may not be able to read these measurements taken by doctors and dentists to measure your ears, eyes, and dental erosion, they do have their own language. Give these providers your records and allow them to communicate with each other on a level we as patients do not need to understand.

Part 17. Dental Healthcare. Keeping track of your medical records is imperative to good health, and just as important is the time and money wasted on redoing dental procedures because a dentist has no records to look at. Keep all your dental records and films in one place. When you go to the dentist, always take your medical records with you. Dentists work and think like physicians in terms of comparing your past dental health to your present-day health. They are not in the profession to pull teeth but to save teeth. They look at prevention versus procedure. Because dental insurance is expensive and not covered by many employers or Medicare, millions of Americans must pay out of pocket for this expense. Abscesses and dental decay cause infections, which then become medical problems. Again, because of the cost, Congress will not justify covering this benefit for 55 million Americans.

Poor dental hygiene also leads to poor nutrition. Folks who can keep their teeth in good repair have a far better chance of a healthier lifestyle, as well as a healthy social life. People who do not have good teeth may be subject to isolation due to embarrassment over their appearance.

Part 18: Hearing. Always keep a record of your hearing tests. With so many people serving in our military these days, guns and loud noises, laborers working near loud machines, ear buds, and our youth with loud music playing on their headsets, hearing is going to be a major issue. Hearing loss can also be caused by medications. Hearing loss is not just about losing parts of conversations; it is also not hearing the phone ring, smoke alarms, car horns, and doorbells. Hearing loss is not an all-or-none disease. We lose our hearing by frequencies. Patients will say they can hear birds. But in truth, they can hear only some of the birds' frequencies, not all of them. Some folks have high-pitched voices. High frequency is the first to go. The elderly will tend to talk to those they can hear and then others wonder why grandma shuns them. The choice is not personal; it lies in the frequency of the voice, pitch, or tone.

There are several things to know about hearing loss. It is documented that hearing loss increases the chances that a person will develop dementia by 60 percent.[4]

Hearing loss is also a major social issue. People who cannot hear tend to isolate themselves in a sea of loneliness and depression because they cannot contribute to conversations. Many people cannot afford the exorbitant price of hearing aids. If they can get hearing aids, many people do not wear them because they are too loud or uncomfortable. Hearing aids take time to adjust to.

Some hearing aids can cost upwards of $10,000 for a set. If you are shopping for hearing aids, it is imperative that you go to a store that sells not on commission but based on the actual cost of the set. This will keep the cost down tremendously. I have seen the same set of hearing aids at Costco for $1,200 and at an audiologist's office for $4,000.

Part 19: Special Issues. No medical chart is complete without this section. Medical issues that loom over us as we age have to be addressed somewhere. These are issues that tend to occur and then leave us alone. Should they arise again in the future, we need to have the records to review in order to remember what treatment worked and what did not. "Special medical issues" are usually kept in a special folder and brought out only if a diagnosis rears itself again. So, what are special issues?

Pregnancy. Here is a perfect example of a medical issue that comes and goes. Should the patient have a high-risk pregnancy but have to find another obstetrician for her next pregnancy, she needs to have her records ready for review. High-risk pregnancies are a valid concern in today's medicine. According to a May 2017 NPR report,[5] the United States has the worst rate of maternal deaths in a developed country. Hospitals are not prepared to handle emergency protocols and there are no standard protocols among obstetricians.

Knowing your risks when giving birth is an important reason to keep your medical records.

Worker's Injury and Compensation. Many employees will suffer a medical mishap while on the job. This is a special issue that must be part of your medical record. Getting your records from the employer's worker's compensation agency can be very difficult. As years go by, the injury may come back in the form of a new problem. Physicians would like to know the cause and treatment of the original injury.

Automobile Accidents. These can be a special issue. When a patient is injured, neck pain or leg pain can be resolved but show up later in life. It is imperative that all films and reports on imaging studies be kept in a special folder under this special issue. This is a huge reference point for physicians who must keep their patients active and social in the years to come.

Special issues can come in many different forms and flavors. Whatever these circumstances are, it is always a good idea to keep records of these debilitating diseases, injuries, or disorders in a folder for easy reference.

Things like *menopause, cancer, dementia, mental health, alcoholism, suicidal tendencies,* and *depression* can be special issues. Do not forget to address these things and keep them separate from the rest of your medical chart in case they arise again. Your family members may be suffering from the same or similar issues. It may be important to pass on your medical chart to them.

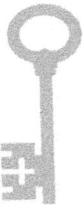

Many patients suffer from depression from time to time. This can be brought on by work, loss of a loved one, divorce, moving, menopause, andropause, surgery, pain medications, changing jobs, or other stressful events or circumstances. Stress and depression seem to be rampant in our culture today. Doctor's have a smorgasbord of medications to help their patients combat the effects of anxiety and depression. What seems to work best for one family member may often work best for another. So your doctor may try a medication that he or she knows works best for someone else in your family. Let your doctor know what medication that is. Keep a record of who is on what medication. Family members need to talk about their medications and not hide them from the rest of the family. This goes back to the family history. It is important that families share what works and what does not.

Part 20. Legal Medical Documents. Tough decisions and choices are part of your medical records. Within the hospital and emergency guidelines, every state has different regulations on which policies they can honor and which ones they can't. For example, say that you live in one state and move to another. Are your DNR (do not resuscitate) order, living will, POLST (provider ordering life-saving treatment), and surrogate or healthcare power of attorney updated and consistent with the laws in the new state where you live? As today's aging population grows, more and more folks are spending six months in warmer climates during the winter and six months in their primary state of residency during the summer months. Since we never know when an emergency will strike, it is best to be prepared for all contingencies. Many advocates will transfer a patient back and forth every six months, keeping their medical records updated as well as keeping the patient in good standing with a primary care physician in both parts of the country. No matter what happens, the advocates always have that patient's back.

Now is the time to get these records together. The original forms can be kept in a safe place, always with an attorney. Copies of these documents should be kept in your medical record book.

A patient had an advocate who insisted on getting the names and numbers of every service her client used. These included things like the dry cleaners, gas station, and auto mechanic. Lawyer, doctors (of course), emergency room preferences, hospital preferences, surgeon preferences, bank, safe deposit locations, as well as family and friends to contact. If anything happened to this patient, this advocate could give this one complete list of names to a designated loved one. Well, the patient had a dog. When she suffered an emergency, she refused to leave her dog and, against medical advice, would not go to the hospital. Needless to say, she was near death when her neighbor found her the next morning. Because of this incident, advocates now keep a list of approved pet-boarding facilities for their clients. This means that if you have a pet, you must have its immunization papers and register the pet with at least three different boarding facilities. Why? Because if one place is full, you must have alternate places to board your animal while you are in the hospital.

Emergency choices are for unknown circumstances, unexpected and unprepared for. Do not be the person who is unprepared. The key is to have all your legal health documents in order and ready to go. Whether you are dying today or just recovering from an illness, it is not an easy process for your friends and family. Make it easy on them. Do not ignore the tough times, decisions, and paperwork that loom ahead for each and every one of us.

Another very important part of emergency care is your medical book. It may mean the difference between life and death. If you dare to take an ambulance ride without your records with you, you risk the cost of life or wallet to get you back to good health.

Some advocates require their clients to have the advocate listed as the emergency contact or put a sticker on the inside of the front door of the home for all EMT personnel to see, stating who the advocate is. This could be a professional advocate or a family member. Keep this name and number on the inside of the door. And don't forget to tell the EMTs where that bag of medications is.

One patient advocate shared with me that she went to the emergency room after being notified by the nursing home that her client had fallen and had a head injury. All the patient needed was suturing over the laceration. But the medical team felt it was important to "run some tests and do a CT scan of the head." The advocate knew her client suffered from dementia and severe anxiety and could not answer questions about her care. The advocate called the health surrogate, her client's son, who lived five hundred miles away. The son spoke personally to the doctor and explained that this particular patient had signed off on forgoing unnecessary tests and had a ten-year history of severe dementia. She did not need further evaluation and it was agreed that she could go back to her nursing home after the sutures had been applied. This saved the patient anxiety, the doctor time, and the family stress.

Part 21. Insurance. This is a moving target. Many folks do not understand their insurance policies. They pay huge premiums, and for what? Insurance companies have raised their rates over the years to a point that Americans can no longer pay them.

Medical costs have risen from 5 percent of the gross national product to 18 percent in the past fifty years. Why such a difference? According to The Balance, the problem lies in lifestyle and government insurance.[6]

While the government tries to keep costs down, diabetes and heart disease occur in 50 percent of our population. At least one out of two people in the United States has one of these diseases. The healthy consumer utilizes less than three percent of healthcare costs while those over sixty-five years old consume over 50 percent yet make up less than 20 percent of the population.

American medical care is very good at saving lives. We see this because many patients come from Canada and other socialized-medicine countries to seek better care but do so at a significant cost.

A patient came in to say she had had an injury while traveling abroad. She found herself in a hospital in Greece for a five-day recovery from this injury. While she was worried about the bill and who was going to pay for it, she soon learned that her total cost for her five-day hospital stay and treatments was $4,200. That's it. She went on to state she got extremely good care and did not feel she missed out on any part of her treatment.

But the opposite can occur. Five hundred million Canadians come south to Florida, Arizona, California, Hawaii, and Texas annually to escape the harsh winter weather up north. They are unprepared for emergencies. When a Canadian citizen has to go to the emergency room, the healthcare system in Canada is notified by the American doctor. Once the patient is stabilized, Canada will send a jet south to pick the patient up and return her or him home in order to reduce the cost of medical bills. They know how expensive American medicine can be.

Therefore, it is imperative that all Americans seek out the insurance they need and can afford. With premiums skyrocketing and deductibles rising higher, few Americans feel comfortable with their cost or their coverage. This is one of the reasons patients are flocking to direct primary care physicians and leaving insurance costs behind. Being able to afford these physicians and working with them is a dream come true for those who want excellent medical care at low costs. This will be discussed further in chapter 14.

Every healthcare advocate has an insurance broker who does not work for an insurance company but works for their clients. They are not paid on commission but are paid by clients to review their insurance plans and find the ones that work best for them. This is an annual review done during the period of open enrollment.

Insurance brokers or patient advocates can also explain the terminology used by insurance companies. Co-pays add up quickly, especially when one is seeing a specialist. Likewise, you have deductibles and out-of-pocket expenses. Then there are the terms "in-network" and "out-of-network." Understand these terms and what you must have in the bank in order to pay your correct bill. We will talk more about billing mistakes in the next chapter.

Many people think physicians and midlevel providers know the cost of the tests they order. Nothing could be further from the truth. The pharmacist does not even know what drugs will cost until the computer spits out a dollar amount. Medical costs are on the dark side of medicine and addressed only when they come out of our bank accounts. Prevention is the mother of invention, which means get the cost out there ahead of time and, except in an emergency, do your homework.

Know what your insurance will and will not pay for. Insurance companies have the right to hide behind the slogan "While you are preapproved, this does not constitute that payment will be made on your behalf." In other words, you may or may not have to pay. Your insurance company is not in business to pay all your bills.

As a family practice physician assistant, it was my job to order appropriate CT or MRI scans for my patients when I felt it was necessary. I would ask my nurse to call the insurance company for preauthorization. Sometimes the representative would say yes and that was fine. Most times, the representative would deny the preauthorization. At this point my nurse would hand me the phone and I would explain to the representative that we were going to end up in a court of law over the death of this patient if she did not give me preapproval. I also required the representative to give me her full name and social security number, so I could find her in five years, when this thing went to trial and she could testify as to why she denied this imaging study. One hundred percent of the time the representative would then say, "Oh look! The computer just said it was preapproved!" Unbelievable that our healthcare system is based on saying no first and then yes. No wonder doctors are leaving the profession. They cannot care for their patients when insurance companies do not care.

Another physician who works in an urgent care facility told me he is the only income generator for the whole clinic. His actions must pay for the lease of the building, the heating, cooling, electricity, and water. His actions also pay for the cost of the electronic medical record system; the salaries for three nurses, two receptionists, and one ex-ray technician; and the cost of the x-ray machine and all the medical supplies needed for the employees to operate safely.

Patients need to realize that they may be paying for bells and whistles but not service. Patients have to ask themselves if they need fresh donuts and coffee in the waiting room or would rather be seen quickly and get care they feel comfortable with. The spectrum of healthcare is broad and diversified. Every office has something to offer someone. It really depends what you are wanting in your healthcare. Being satisfied with your doctor means different things to different people. Being safe within the system means the same thing to all of us.

A doctor went to Canada on vacation. While he was there his wife got very ill. He took her to the emergency room at a local hospital. When they arrived, she went straight into the exam room and was seen and stabilized. After an hour of waiting, this doctor peeked his head out and saw all employees sitting around a desk. He asked what was going on. They all looked at their watches and then one said, "You came in at the end of the shift and we have run out of Canadian Healthcare money. We are waiting for the next shift to begin and then you will be seen for further treatment. This is when the next shift of money starts. We are allowed to see patients only until the money runs out, and then we stop appointments and procedures. If your wife was not able to be stabilized, we would continue care, but at this point we need to wait."

So this may explain why many Canadians have their own medical brokers who find them ways to get procedures done faster in the United States than in Canada. If you have to wait twelve months to get a knee replaced because they are booking that far ahead based on high numbers of patients, it makes sense to go elsewhere if you have the money.

Get with your insurance broker or healthcare advocate to lower the costs of your medications, as well as to study your insurance plan and know what it involves. These folks are experts at deciphering the chaos found in the insurance policy of Smoke and Mirrors.

Part 22. Medical Bills. Don't pay that bill. Speaking of smoke and mirrors, it is amazing that patients pay medical bills. Why Americans will spend countless hours looking for a great deal on Amazon and then pay a medical bill without verifying the contents, cost, and accuracy is beyond comprehension.

Many patients will pay in response to the "Explanation of Benefits" even when it says it huge letters not to pay that bill. If all patients started looking at their medical bills like they do their cell phone bills, the healthcare industry would clean up their billing methods and have to be held accountable to you, the customer, the patient.

We will address more of this in chapter 11.

CHAPTER 9

What You Should Know When Your Doctor Gives You Orders

L et's talk about all the extras your doctor can order for you. In chapter 4, we talked about the Plan — part 4 of the SOAP note. What is your doctor asking you to do? Collectively, we call these *medical extras*. These include things like labs — and there are hundreds of different blood labs we could do. Cultures can be anything that comes out of the body and grows bacteria, fungi, or viruses. If we can get a swab of it and put it in a Petri dish, we can culture it and see what kind of nuisance is growing out of it. Then we will also look at imaging. Imaging studies encompass x-rays, ultrasound, MRIs, CT scans, bone density scans, PET scans, and many more. Other medical extras include services such as treatment by specialists, physical therapy, home health, or perhaps chiropractic medicine. We could also refer you for either acupuncture, homeopathic medicine, or other alternative medicine such as Active Release Therapy. Providers can also refer you to a patient advocate, who is going to take care of you and oversee and coordinate all your medical treatment. Then the provider may also order supplies — anything from dietary food to adult diapers to oxygen, nebulizers, walkers, wheelchairs, compression stockings, sleep apnea machines, or canes. All you have to do is walk into a medical supply store to see that the list is endless, including even electric recliner chairs, special portable toilet seats, and hospital beds.

Moving forward, there are three questions you always want to ask your doctor no matter what the doctor orders.

1) *What are you looking for?* In other words, what are you thinking? Have you formulated any ideas as to what the diagnosis could be? Why are you ordering this? What are you looking to find by ordering this?

2) *What is the worst this could be?* This question makes the provider stop and think. Providers will usually ask themselves, "Am I missing anything?" "Is this as serious as I am making it out to be?"

3) *What will our next plan be if the tests come back normal?* This makes your provider stop and think what the next plan of action will be if your plan results in no solution.

Let's look at an example of how this might work. Many patients will go through tests that find nothing, though the patient still has the pain. Worse, the pain is now in the patient's wallet, too. If pain is an issue, then the doctor is ordering a test or service to try to discover the origin of the pain. If the test result is normal, then what?

A patient came in one day with her advocate. As we went through steps 3 through 6, the advocate took notes. As I discussed her plan, her three questions came up.

I had ordered an MRI on this patient's knee.

What are you looking for? Torn ligaments, arthritis, or bone spurs, I answered.

What is the worst it could be? A lot of arthritis and possibly a knee replacement in the near future, I said.

What will you recommend if the test is normal? Physical therapy or perhaps rest and anti-inflammatory medications, I explained.

The patient then spoke up and said, "Since the MRI is going to cost me a $400 deductible, can I do the physical therapy, rest, and ibuprofen first? If the knee is not better (or gets worse), can we then do the MRI?" This is a very valid point, well taken. Providers are not in business to cost their patients money. Cost should always be a major concern. We now had a plan, expectations, and an agreement about what might work best for the patient now.

Let's examine two more big rules about orders:

Always get the name of the report — this means that every report, order, or imaging study must have a name at the top of the report. You can find this name on the report to be sure it is the same name you wrote down when you left the doctor's office. Many times a doctor will order a type of test, and when the patient gets to the lab or x-ray machine, the radiologist wants to order another one.

I have seen different doctor's order the same labs over and over again for the same patient. I have also seen incorrect mammograms and sonograms done because a test was not looking for the right things or was not in the right area.

Always get a copy of the report. Get the results and keep them in a folder until you can see your doctor again and have the doctor look them over. Never think that "normal" means okay. You must always get a copy of your report. A missed report can be a deadly report until someone reads it.

Labs

Lab costs are in the billions of dollars every year. Five billion tests are ordered each year; imagine how much money is spent. Thirty percent of all labs are unnecessary. There are certainly ways for you to prevent this. The wrong blood labs are ordered 30 percent of the time. And this is something that also has to be addressed. This means 15 million tests, each year in the United States, that did not tell the physician what he or she wanted to know. The patient and the insurance company had to pay the bill for the wrong test. Why are so many wrong tests ordered? Many of the errors are related to the wrong tube, method used to draw the blood, or storage for the blood.

Then there are certain medications that can alter the results of a lab. There are results that can show disease when there is none or miss disease that is there.

How accurate are labs? It depends. No labs are 100 percent, because of the human factor of how and when a sample is collected. But every lab has a *sensitivity* and *specificity*. Sensitivity means that if the test is highly sensitive and the result is negative (normal), then you can be fairly certain you do not have that disease. Specificity means that if the test is highly specific and the result is positive (abnormal), you can be fairly certain that you have the disease. Make sure you cover these two topics with your doctor before your labs are ordered.

So why do providers order exams or tests that are unnecessary? What are they looking for? There are several different answers here. It really depends on the patient. You should always ask the very specific question "What are you looking for in this test?" And write down the answer. When the provider can't answer it, then you've got a problem. It is important for the provider to give you an answer to this question. Many times providers will say, "Well, let's wait and see what the tests say and then we'll have you back again." Well, what if the tests are normal and you still have the pain? Where do you go from there?

Here are few rules of the road about labs. Your insurance plan does not cover all labs. You have to check with your ordering physician about which ones you need, and you have to be sure the diagnosis code is correct in order for the test to be covered. Never get labs done until you know the prices and coverage. Ask about the blood draw. This could be expensive as well. What do these labs charge just to stick a needle in your arm? In some offices, the cost to draw blood and then ship it out is another $50 to $60 added to your bill. But if you went to the lab directly and got your blood drawn, there wouldn't be any charge and they might even use the correct tube to draw the blood. Multiple tests like lipid panels or thyroid panels may be charged for each test within the panel. Average lab tests are $460 out of your pocket. They are expensive, and the best way to handle such an expense is to call your insurance company to find out where you can get these labs and what they cost. Your provider does not know these costs but should know why they are ordering the lab tests and what the correct diagnostic code is.

Asking the above three questions every time your provider orders a test will cover all your concerns and costs.

Preventive Labs

Okay, so let's say you've called the insurance company and you've gone to the right lab and you're having blood drawn for your annual checkup. If these tests are coded for "preventive medicine," then your insurance will pay them. But oftentimes providers just don't know what codes to use for what labs, and if they're not covered then you're going to end up paying out of pocket.

Make sure that your provider knows that he or she is using the correct code, so you won't have to pay for these labs. Go to the lab if it's cheaper to draw blood there. Find out which labs are in your network. Lab tests are never emergencies unless you are in the emergency room. You have time to get your lab work done. Don't just go where it's convenient. Convenience can cost you hundreds of dollars more.

One client kept getting a bill for $300 for her mammogram. We knew it should fall under preventive care. The first and second times we called her insurance company they said they would send the bill back to the physician's office and fix it. When we got a third bill and called the insurance company, the woman on the phone told us she had "pushed a button" and said, "All fixed!" We never did figure out who was supposed to have "pushed the button" — the doctor or the insurance representative.

Specimens

A "specimen" is a fluid or tissue sample that has been removed from you. It can be any solid, liquid, or gas taken out of your body for examination. Gases could come from your lungs, the solid could come from your skin or your liver, and the liquid could be your blood, stool, or urine. A "biopsy" is examination of tissue for abnormal growth by a pathologist. The pathologist looks at the tissue under a microscope to identify good tissue versus bad tissue, such as cancer cells.

A "culture" is something that takes time to grow and analyze in the lab. An example of a culture would be a urine culture, where the lab is looking to see if bacteria grow and identify which kind they are.

Lab Test Panels

A set of tests that are normally ordered together is a "panel." These labs are grouped together to make it easier for the physician to order and not forget an important lab. Panels also tend to include similar tests that, when their results are considered together, will give the doctor a better picture of your diagnosis.

There are also other types of tests that may or may not be done in the doctor's office: the strep test, the flu test, the mono test. Even though these are fairly easy tests to do and are ordered fairly frequently, check their accuracy and whether you really need them. Some of them are very expensive. One common question a physician will often ask her- or himself is, "Will the results of the test change how I am going to treat the patient?" If the answer is no, then do you really need the test?

Imaging

When we talk about imaging studies, we are talking about everything from taking a picture to taking a peek — in other words, x-rays, CT scans, MRIs, nerve conduction studies, EKGs, gastrointestinal (GI) scopes, colonoscopies. Imaging studies include any time someone takes a picture of you, sticks a tube or an instrument in you, or puts you on the table and scans you or does any kind of invasive test. Even pulmonary function tests could go under imaging studies. What you want to do is make sure you write down the name of the test when you get your report back — and you must always request that a report be sent to you. Know that your physician has to review the report first before releasing it to you. While this means someone looks at it, I have seen more and more scribes and nurses, instead of the doctor, reading these reports. This can lead to medical error.

Another thing I want to mention is that when a radiologist or pathologist gives us a report, they put in the body of the report what they are seeing and observing. And then on the bottom of the report they put the "impression." I was taught early in my career to read both — never just read the impression. And I believe most providers follow this same rule. I have actually seen in the body of a report that there was a cancerous growth and yet the impression said that everything was normal. So I have had to notify the radiologist to please reread the test and issue another report. This report can be read easily by any physician, and a second set of eyes is the safety factor needed in a sea of mistakes. Keep this report with you and file it only after you have had your physician or even two physicians review it with you. You do not need to make a special trip to the doctor's office. Depending on how you doctor works, you can drop a copy off at the office or email it, and the doctor will look at it.

The lab or the facility that does the report has to send it back to your provider. If it is preauthorized, the provider's office has called and gotten the authorization from the patient's insurance company that they will pay for this test. However, it is known that they often only say that they will pay for it — this doesn't mean they actually will pay for it. They say they are preauthorizing it though, based on final evaluation, they will determine whether or not to pay for it at all. So you need to know that the patient is sometimes stuck with the bill even though it was preauthorized. We'll talk about how to handle bills like these in module seven. Just always get a preauthorization; make sure it's been done, and oftentimes they'll even give you a confirmation or preauthorization number. To make sure this has been done correctly, not only do you need that code number, but the doctor has to code correctly for this test to be done

X-Rays

Most of us are familiar with x-rays. They may be done in a provider's office as well as in an emergency room or hospital. They are even done in urgent treatment centers or convenient care centers. Providers are looking for bones — broken bones. They look for objects that you may have swallowed, pneumonia, foreign objects that may be found in cuts. You also get x-rays when you have mammograms; CT scans do that too. If you are going to get an x-ray read, by your provider if you are in an office or an emergency room, the provider will tell you what the x-ray says; however, because these x-rays also have to be read — just like CT scans or MRI's — by a radiologist, expect to see that bill as well.

MRIs

MRIs are interesting. This diagnostic tool does not use radiation, so it's relatively safe. It can even be used on pregnant women, although it's not recommended in the first three months. But everybody does a case-by-case study to see if the MRI is a good tool to use or not. MRIs are used to look at blood vessels and abnormal tissues and breasts and bones and joints, including knee replacements and so on. MRIs are also a good idea when you are looking for the difference between Alzheimer's disease and some other form of dementia. MRIs have also been known to catch a stroke early so that the patient can be given anticoagulants before the stroke gets worse. MRIs are always good for looking at the brain or when you need to see a lot of detail. Unfortunately, MRIs are really expensive, but if you shop around you'll be shocked at the differences in price. We will talk more about this in chapter 11 on financial responsibility.

Pet Scans

Positron emission thermography, known as a PET scan, involves radiation as well, just like CT scans and x-rays. However, the radiation in a PET scan is just a radioactive tracer that's put in your system ahead of time.

PET scans can be combined with CT scans to get a complete picture of what your body looks like and what kinds of diseases there may be. This option is very effective in diagnosing neurological diseases like multiple sclerosis and Alzheimer's.

Also, for cancer, PET scans can be used to assess effectiveness of treatment. They detect cancers — brain, breast, cervical, colorectal, esophageal, head, neck, lung, lymphoma, melanoma, pancreatic, prostate, thyroid — all of these. Cancer cells actually show up as bright spots on the PET scan because they have a higher metabolic rate than normal cells.

PET scans can also be used in the assessment of heart conditions — helping your doctor decide which arteries are clogged — and brain disorders. They can differentiate between tumors, Alzheimer's, and seizures.

But this is a diagnostic tool — it is not going to fix anything. And again, you always have to ask your provider, "Why are you doing this? What are you going to do with the results?"

Ultrasounds

Most of us are familiar with ultrasounds. They are used commonly with pregnant women to see how the baby is doing, including checking the baby's heart. They are basically soundwaves that bounce off internal objects and produce images. We can look at an abnormal heart or at a patient's blood vessels, ovaries, uterus, or testicles.

Ultrasounds are also used quite commonly in sickle-cell anemia to find abdominal abnormalities in such organs as the liver, gallbladder, spleen, or kidneys. They work great for breast cancer because they can actually guide the fine-needle aspiration when a doctor is trying to take a biopsy of certain cells in a mass in the breast. Ultrasounds are also good for rheumatic conditions. People with rheumatic arthritis have actually had their medications changed when doctors have seen how certain medications have worked and others have not, based on ultrasound images of those joints. So ultrasound is a very handy tool to have. Ultrasound is used quite frequently in emergency rooms to assess trauma of the human body; it can save lives. When a victim of a motor-vehicle accident comes in and the doctor just doesn't even know where to begin, the doctor can safely use ultrasound to examine the whole body.

Preparations

Be prepared for your test. It may be extremely hard to find the right person to ask about your test. Do you need to drink water before the test, or empty your bladder? Do you eat before the test or avoid food for eight hours? Your ordering doctor usually has a paper with instructions on it about your test. If not, ask for the instructions but make sure the person you ask knows the answer. If you're not sure, have the person call the radiology technician to learn the answer. Too many patients have been told not to eat for eight hours before a test only to find out they could have eaten regular meals all the way up to the test.

Another aspect for which you will need to prepare is cost. After you have discerned why your provider is ordering the test, what the prep involves, and what your physician is going to do with the results, it is time to look at cost. You have to call your insurance company and find out who is going to cover this. If the insurance company agrees to pay for the test, make sure they are also agreeing to cover the radiologist or pathologist who has to read the image or tissue. If the answer is yes, then the next question should be, "Is this radiologist or pathologist in or out of my network?" Many patients have had their imaging and surgeries done in-network only to find out the radiologist or pathologist was out of network.

And, likewise, as with labs and cultures, you must always get a report of your imaging study. At the very top of the report, it will tell you what kind of report it is.

Services

Any time you have to have a service related to medical treatment, medical home health, or nonmedical, you are going to have to get a copy of the report. Because insurance pays for services based on their reports, you must have reports for all of them. Ask for a copy of it. And again, you are going to put it in this section, with the date(s) of service. For example, you have physical therapy ordered three times a week. Why? Because you hurt your shoulder. And then success? Yes, it was fixed. So, the question here is, how many times have you gone in or the provider (like myself) has seen a patient and said, "Your shoulder hurts. Okay. Have you ever had this problem before?" "Yes, I did." "Well what did you do about it?" "Well I had physical therapy." "How did that work?" "I guess okay. I'm not really sure." "Okay. Well, who was it?" "Oh, it was this fabulous person in physical therapy. I absolutely loved the person that did it." "Do you remember their name?" "No." This time you will. Why? Because you can go back to this physical therapy report and find name of the excellent physical therapist again. You can do the same with surgeons, specialists, nurses, and anyone else who helped you and to whom you want to go back again for more services. You are not going to lose your good providers.

CHAPTER 10

Your Legal Responsibility in Healthcare

The Unknowns, Unexpecteds, and Emergencies

When that ambulance is backing up to the emergency door and the patient is coming in on a gurney, the first thing the nurse will ask is, "What's wrong with the patient?" The emergency medical personnel — the EMTs — will try as hard as they can to give the nurse a description.

One day a patient was rolled into the ER. He was probably in his eighties. He was unconscious, and the EMTs had no information on him. I asked them, "What's wrong with him?" And they said, "We don't know. We just found him on the floor at the nursing home and nobody seemed to know what was wrong." I asked if anyone had any medical background on this patient and they said no. So I picked up the phone and called the nursing home that he came from and I said to the person on the phone, "Can you tell me about Mr. So-and-so?" And her response was, "Oh, is he not in his room?" I was shocked and so was she. When she realized that I was calling from the emergency room and that he'd been picked up by an ambulance, she said to hold on a minute, now becoming embarrassed, and went to get someone on the phone. In the meantime, is the patient was losing precious seconds when I could be treating him. I didn't know why he'd passed out. I didn't know if he had hit his head. Again, I had no information on him.

Change up the scenario a little bit. Let's say I have this patient and he comes rolling in on the gurney, and he's unconscious but I find the Patient's Medical History Book on his stomach, or better yet, I have a patient advocate standing there with him saying, "I know everything you need to know about Mr. Smith. His adult children live out-of-state and I take care of him. The nursing home called me. Let me tell you everything about his condition and why, most probably, he is like this. I also have all his legal papers in case he starts to fail. And I have all his contacts." Imagine the time and money that are going to be saved and the tests I won't have to do because I have that kind of information. It is powerful!

Your Patient Rights

The details of your rights as a patient are defined in the Emergency Medical Treatment and Active Labor Act (EMTALA) laws in the United States. Many people think that patient rights are applicable only between themselves and their doctor. This is not the case; patient rights can be extensive and exist between many people and institutions. Most notably, they can exist between patients and any medical caregiver, hospitals, laboratories, insurers, and even secretarial help and housekeepers that may have access to patients or their medical records.

Every healthcare institution has some form of patient rights and you should see, read, and understand them. Below is an example.

"All patients should be guaranteed the following freedoms:

→ To seek consultation with the physician(s) of their choice;
→ To know the identity of those who treat them;
→ To be treated with courtesy and respect;
→ To contract with their physician(s) on mutually agreeable terms;

→ To be treated confidentially, with access to their records limited to those involved in their care or designated by the patient;

→ To use their own resources to purchase the care of their choice;

→ To refuse medical treatment even if it is recommended by their physician(s);

→ To be relieved of pain;

→ To be informed about their medical condition, the risks and benefits of treatment, and appropriate alternatives;

→ To refuse third-party interference in their medical care, and to be confident that their actions in seeking or declining medical care will not result in third-party-imposed penalties for patients or physicians;

→ To be given privacy;

→ To receive full disclosure of their insurance plan language;

→ To be given full counseling upon request;

→ To receive an estimate of charges of medical care; and

→ To give informed consent.

There are no set rules regarding patient's rights. Everyone uses their own interpretations.

"Health directives" is an umbrella term that really encompasses three parts.

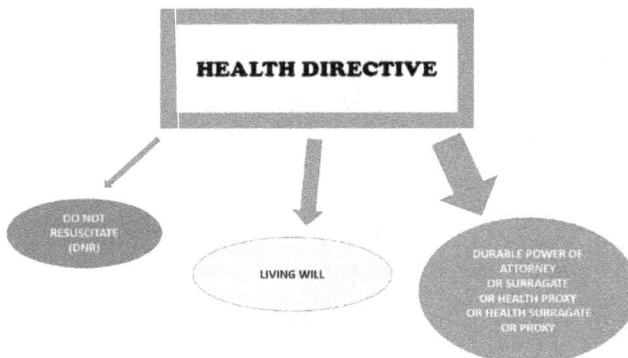

The first document, titled "Do Not Resuscitate" (DNR), is really not a very comprehensive way of telling anyone in the healthcare profession what you want. It basically says that if your heart stops beating, you do not want to be revived with cardiopulmonary resuscitation, also known as CPR. That is pretty simple.

The next question is, if you are comatose or cannot speak for yourself (the yellow part above), your living will can tell us what you want us to do. This gets very tricky because every state and every doctor and nurse can interpret this information differently.

A patient advocate is sometimes hired by the client to go to an attorney's office and set up all the legal documentation to provide for the time when the client can no longer speak for him- or herself. One client's attorney told me never to have a living will. When I asked why, she explained that her client had pneumonia and, because the client had a living will that instructed that treatment be withheld, he died. She said antibiotics could have saved him and he would have made a full recovery. I then met with another client's attorney. When we got to the living will, I stated my concerns against having one. She corrected me and stated that a living will is designed to address only mechanical life-support machines and not antibiotics or other treatment. Since both attorneys practiced within the same state, I was confused.

Upon digging deeper, I realized that the interpretation of the living will is left up to the doctor or nurse, who truly does not want this kind of responsibility. Nor are they educated in living will documents. Therefore, an advocate, family member, or professional must always be familiar with the patient's wishes and keep on top of treatment plans.

So a living will really doesn't give us specifics that we need, but the durable power of attorney does. This is also known as the health proxy or the surrogate or the person who tells us exactly what the loved one said. That they might want antibiotics if they could have a full recovery. That they might want oxygen if it was needed. That they would like surgery. An interesting example of this might be about a doctor stopping in the middle of surgery, coming out and saying to the family, "I've reached the point here where I can go further, but I'm not sure the patient is going to have the quality of life she wants. What do you want me to do?" And the family knows exactly what the patient would be happy with. And they say, "As long as she can continue to see, visit, and speak with family and loved ones, that's all she is asking for." It doesn't matter whether she has to stay bedridden; it doesn't matter if she can't walk; it doesn't matter if she can't use the restroom anymore but has to be confined to the bed. Her only wish is that she can see and speak to her loved ones and enjoy their company. This is her wish.

So let's go back to living wills, because it's important, especially for people who live in the north but come south or to a warmer climate every winter, to know that there are different regulations and rules in every single state — different laws. With every state having different legal requirements in terms of how many people must sign the document and what is or is not included in the living will, it is best practice to have a *health surrogate* designated who can speak for you no matter where you are.

I have seen patients die when their wishes were ignored. One patient's doctor was ready to do a liver transplant and could have given him many more years. The patient had excellent health otherwise. His liver failed due to cancer. His estranged wife moved him into hospice, and he passed five days later. His advocate and children knew he had wanted a liver transplant. He just never designated a legal health surrogate, so his estranged wife oversaw his legal affairs.

Many states are adopting POLST-like documents. This stands for "provider ordering life sustaining-treatment." It involves a conversation between patient and physician in which the patient's wishes are spelled out. Once the provider and patient sign this document, it becomes legally binding. This is important in that it means family members cannot change or vacillate on decisions about their loved one. They are already emotionally distraught, so this document relieves them of the burden of decision. Medical personnel must follow the instructions in this document, since it is now a statute attached to the life of the patient. It contains a very clear and concise directive as to what the patient wants done. Once it is signed by patient and provider, no one can change it but the patient.

When you have a health surrogate, you must have a conversation with that person about your quality of life. Do not leave them to decide for you. I know many health surrogates who will not agree to the responsibility unless the patient states exactly what he or she can or cannot live with.

Many professional patient advocates will meet their clients in the emergency room. Before this happens, the most advanced, better-trained patient advocates have prepared their clients for emergencies.

Where should you keep your legal healthcare papers?

Depending on what state you live in, the answer to the question above will vary. If you are in a POLST-statute state, your POLST document should be posted on your refrigerator. EMTs will know to look for it there.

The key is to keep the document with one person; do not make multiple copies. Make sure one person is in charge of it. This person needs to know who your health surrogate is. You must destroy any older copies of the document so there is no confusion. Many times a patient will tell one family member one thing and another family member something else. It is imperative that all people involved work together.

> I had a mom who was terminal and told her daughter about her cancer and asked her to "let her go" when the time was right. She did not tell her son about her cancer, as she did not want to "worry him." When the patient was hospitalized in her final days and the daughter spoke up about doing the least possible, the son was distraught. It was then that the sister had to tell her brother the sorrowful news. He picked up the hospital chair and threw it across the room out of anguish. It is unfair to put this burden on one person without giving this person the support they are going to need from all others who care too.

CHAPTER 11

Your Financial Responsibility in Healthcare

Why are healthcare costs now the number one cause of bankruptcy in America today? There are several factors involved. Let's look at a few.

Ridiculously high cost of materials and services

No one will dispute the fact that businesses have to make money to stay in business. Now that we have accepted the fact that healthcare is a business, how do we separate this from the cash-pay doctors? High medical bills are driven by the high cost of all products and services in healthcare. We have all heard that a bag of sterile water can cost $400. If this same sterile water was sold in a grocery store, then the cost might be $4.00, because the consumer would not pay for it otherwise.

Before I became a physician assistant, I did not know how confusing the healthcare system was. One day I went to see a gastroenterologist who was a friend of mine. Her office sent a bill for $400. Then I received an "explanation of benefits" in the mail. It showed that the insurance would pay $120. I had already paid my deductible. I called my friend and asked her if I could pay her the difference, since she wasn't getting the total amount she was charging. She explained to me that this is a game physicians play with insurance. Insurances pay a "percentage" of the bill, never the whole bill. So, for her to get the $120 for an office visit, she needed to charge $400. She said to not worry about it. It just seemed so odd that something like this occurred.

Can you imagine getting your cell phone bill, calling the company and telling them you will only pay 30 percent of it? How does insurance get away with this? Why not make these bills transparent for all to see and everyone pay 100 percent of the agreed price?

Third-party payers — "Oh, my insurance will cover it and I deserve it."

In an earlier example, you saw a patient who knew that her deductible for an MRI was going to be $400. She wanted to hold off on incurring such a charge until she needed to. Most patients are not this astute. Doctors hear patients everyday say, "Insurance will pay for it." And this drives the cost up for everyone. The doctor's order is not an emergency and patients should truly look around for lower costs, because in the end, everyone is paying for insurance. You should take the time to call your insurance company and find out where you should go to get your imaging study or labs done at the lowest cost. Since these tests are not emergencies, many patients find the time to check with friends and neighbors about the best places to go and get the best services.

Even better yet is the patient advocate, who knows where to go to get the MRI because the cost will be the lowest. It

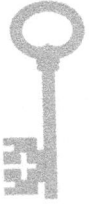

is always a good idea to ask the patient advocate for at least three places to go before deciding. Another key is to be sure to confirm that the amount quoted includes the radiologist's bill to read the MRI, x-ray, or other imaging study. You do not want to get another bill unexpectedly for $100 to $200 more.

As a Patient Best advocate, I will shop around for my clients. Most of my clients have a deductible that they have to pay regardless of the total cost. Then they have coinsurance, too. This is usually 20 percent of the remaining bill. Let's do the math. In the different areas I've worked and practiced medicine, every town had a really cheap MRI scan that could be done for $300; an MRI scan done in the hospital is usually $2500.

Twenty percent of $300 means a $60 coinsurance payment and 20 percent of $2500 means a $500 coinsurance payment. There is no difference in the machines and radiologists. Both have to qualify to perform the service safely and effectively. So there can be a huge difference in the prices for the same imaging study.

So shop around; start looking at the different areas in your town that offer imaging studies and see who does them for less. It may still be cheaper for you to go to a place out of network than to a place your insurance company wants you to go to.

More and more patients are moving toward these less expensive medical practices and procedures and not paying

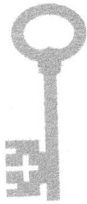

insurance at all. Insurance rates are so high now, deductibles are ridiculously high, and then the cost of services is still higher, and patients are stuck with heavy bills. Many patients are now turning to direct primary care physicians (see chapter 14). Then, if they need extra services, they are being directed where to get their labs and studies done. They pay for that one service and do not need to worry about monthly insurance premiums anymore. They pay for a service and move on — one and done.

I don't know the cost, but I will order it anyway.

One patient came in the office with a cut on her finger. Because it was only oozing, it was treated with cauterization (burning). The diagnosis was laceration. Unbeknownst to the physician, a diagnosis of "laceration" came with a $350 suture kit as well as a $125 office-visit charge. When the patient went to check out, she had no insurance. She had to pay $425 for a fifteen-minute visit to cauterize a wound. The receptionist felt sorry for the patient and asked the doctor about this. The doctor was mortified that this cost was so high. She spent the next twenty minutes hitting different diagnosis buttons on her computer while the receptionist told her what the cost was from her computer. She could not look cost up on her computer, but the receptionist had access to the cost sheets. Fragmented systems do this. Finally, they arrived at a cost of $50 for the patient to pay and filed it under wound care. If the patient had had insurance, this incorrect bill would have charged her insurance $425 for a suture kit she never used.

Besides the bill overcharging on materials you never received, there is also the unjustified expectation that the bill should be paid even though medical error has occurred. Doctors are not at fault, as they rarely ever know the cost of any services or products.

I'll just pay the bill.

With medical bills being wrong over 90 percent of the time, why is it that patients continue to pay them? One answer lies in the patient who feels she or he got a deal.

> One patient (actually a physician) who had prostate cancer finished his treatment regimen, which included prostate removal and post-operational surgical care. He got a bill from the hospital for $46,000. His insurance paid all but $3600. He felt this was a good deal and wanted to pay it. Someone suggested he look over the bill or hire a patient advocate to do it for him. He took their advice, and when he got the final bill, it was $600. His bill was reduced by $3000 and his advocate service was only $900 (30 percent of the amount he saved), so he still saved $2,100.

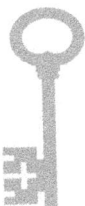

> Never pay a medical bill. Get a patient advocate who specializes in this field and have them look over your bill first, get it corrected, and then pay it. Every advocate charges differently, so discuss fees with the advocate you choose. Knowing you are paying the correct bill gives you such peace of mind. If you hire a tax accountant to do your taxes, why wouldn't you hire a patient advocate to do your medical bills? It is hoped you will not need to file bankruptcy.

Doctors are paid on commission.

> There are thousands of stories about how bad medical bills are. While there are some doctors who will up-charge patients for services they didn't do, most doctors know that

fraud comes with severe punishment and will not be toler-
ated by the US government. Therefore, more people must
be on payroll to ensure this does not happen. This increases
your cost as well.

One has to be careful about billing accuracy. One woman
told me she can no longer get foot care at her assisted living
facility. The podiatrist that comes in once a week had his
office call her and tell her he is all booked up on his days to
her facility. Why? Because when she got her bill, she noticed
that he was charging Medicare for surgery on her foot when
he had done no such thing. He had only clipped her toenails
that day. When she called his office to ask him to change it,
he did, saying it was a medical error but he will no longer
treat her. So much for access to care.

One patient stayed three extra days in the hospital because of a medical error. The hospital wanted him to pay for
the stay. He refused and won that case.

Another patient had a bad outcome from his doctor and
ended up with no follow-up care and refused to pay for
something he did not get.

Many patients will say, "I have good insurance." And those patients are
often the ones who incur the most healthcare expenses. When hospitals
see "good insurance," they know they can charge for services, so they start
sending in multiple doctors to you for consultations while you are in the
hospital. They order more tests and procedures on you than on another
patient who doesn't have "good insurance." You are poked prodded and
stuck with needles more than the average patient. When these "good
insurance" patients get out of the hospital, they have huge coinsurance
bills to pay.

I was working as a patient advocate for one of my clients. Because I teach them and their families to always get the name and number of anyone who comes into the room, they did. On one such occasion, my client had excellent insurance, which meant the hospital administration would want to do excessive consultations and tests on this patient. Along came a doctor who introduced herself as a gerontologist, to check the patient, my client, for dementia. This was not a working diagnosis. Had my client been on mind-altering medications or pain killers, she might have appeared to have dementia or failure to thrive, or been unconscious. Fortunately, my client did not take any such medications. The doctor said she was ordered to evaluate the patient for dementia while she was there getting a knee replacement. Because the patient refused the service, the doctor left. The hospital still billed $450 for a consulting fee, which we had removed.

Medical bills are always wrong, for one or both of two very big reasons:

1. The doctor's office, the hospital cost, and the materials and procedures used and billed to you are grouped together and somehow hidden behind a radio button on the physician's computer. When that button is pressed it generates a cost to the patient and insurance company. Because doctors do not know what is being charged, it's hard for them to know whether a suture tray, a 10-ml syringe, a medication, or whatever was added into that bill. As more and more advocates are finding, bills are incorrect and need to be assessed for accuracy. Finding the hidden costs in a "bundled" bill is a tedious job and most patients do not know where to begin.

Going out to eat at a nice restaurant, most people will check their bill. Upon checking out of a nice hotel, most people will check their bill.

So why do patients not check their bill? Very simple. They are not the ones paying the whole bill. Oftentimes a patient will say that insurance is paying it. This is not the case. Ultimately, the cost is found in premiums and comes right back to the patient. If employees are traveling on company time, they know their employer is paying for it, so they are not concerned about a bill. When you pay for it yourself, you should be very concerned. This is why it is imperative that you know what the bill is for, whether in fact you had the treatment, and what diagnosis tags that bill as acceptable.

2. The medical billing code is wrong. Hospital and large healthcare facilities hire a whole department of coders to be sure bills will get reimbursed by insurance companies. If the doctor does not code correctly, insurance will not pay, and the patient will get stuck with the bill. This occurs a lot when the service is supposed to be coded under preventive services and the insurance is supposed to pay the bill 100 percent. Because of the wrong code, the patient gets the bill. There are many cases like this.

Insurance companies do not like to pay.

Let's look at the other side of this. As mentioned before, more and more physicians are moving to direct primary care. One direct primary care physician told me she moved into her practice because she lost $125,000 in payment the previous year when insurance refused to pay her claims. She said that if she was going to work for free, she might as well not fill out paperwork, too.

Also, if she practices outside the insurance system, she can cut her overhead costs from 65 percent to less than 10 percent every month. Therefore, she does not have to charge the patient so much to keep a biller, electronic medical records, three nurses, paperwork, and so on. She now draws her own blood and has one secretary; patients pay her a monthly fee. Because she does not have so many employees and regulations, she can now see her patients for forty-five minutes to an hour at a time and not worry about paying a huge staff.

Recently one physician told me his patient, who works for a large insurance company, told him that she deals with his office visit charges when he sends them in. She told him that she has to deny most of them and hold the few she will authorize for payment until the very last minute. When he resubmits the denied claims for payment, she told him they go in the garbage two more times. Then on the third try, they may pay him.

So not only is the American public going bankrupt, so is the solo-practice physician who wanted to own his or her own practice someday and spend time with patients, like in the good old days. They cannot keep their doors open and expect insurance to pay.

The American public would do well to keep updated on the movement in Washington, DC, to do away with direct primary care offices. They are a threat to big business. Most recently, lobbyists against direct primary care physicians have offered a hybrid model that is still bad for medical practices and patients. The Center for Medicare and Medicaid (CMS) is looking into paying direct primary care physicians. The problem is that they will still avoid payments, convolute the system, and confuse the patient. It will end up a costly mistake for the American people who want easy, direct care.

PART 3

Why No One Can Walk in Your Shoes

The last part of this book may be the most critical for you. Sure, you have now learned all you need to know to successfully navigate the healthcare system, but there comes a time when we are all too sick or too tired to do it on our own. We must turn to someone for help.

As moms and dads, we have

→ Children to worry about

→ School and homework

→ Dinners to get

As employers and employees, we have

→ Careers to worry about

→ Financial responsibilities

→ Bills to pay

→ No time to take off to be ill

As spouses, we have

→ Marriages to keep intact

→ Communication barriers to overcome

As we age, we may suffer the following losses or changes:

→ Loss of a job

→ Loss of a hobby — golf, playing piano, painting, reading, etc.

→ Loss of a spouse or partner or friends

→ Loss of a home

→ Driver's license — gone

→ Loss of financial control / checkbook

→ Hairdresser — can't get there.

→ Letters from friends — diminishing

→ Sight — slowly going blind

→ Hearing — Where are my expensive hearing aids?

→ Pain — creeping up

→ Medications that make you feel weird, tired, or nauseated

→ Energy — less with every day

→ Pet — died or you can't take care of it

→ Cell phone — can't see the numbers

→ Necklace — traded in for life-line button

→ High heels — to foot solutions with insoles

→ Jewelry — can't wear anymore

→ Places — can't go too far without a bathroom

→ Children — dying before us

→ Loss of social life — leading to depression and sadness

→ Church — can't get there, no ride

→ Shopping — can't leave the bathroom

→ Food — has no taste

Living well takes energy. Getting up every day takes courage. Courage takes energy. It is energy that gives us life. We all have our good days and our bad days.

How do I protect myself from this depletion of energy and well-being? We will give you three options. Pick one or a combination of them to get you through the best years of your life. (care coordinator, family, and/or direct primary care). Let's look at the professional help first and then discuss the son or daughter option, and then the direct primary care physician. Consider the following questions:

→ Why do you need professional support?

→ Why does family not always make for the best assistance?

→ Why drown in your last years when you can swim?

Baby boomers are a generation of Americans born between 1946 and 1964. Eleven thousand baby boomers will turn sixty-five each day from 2011 to 2029. We are currently in the throes of a large portion of our population not only leaving the work force to retire but also using Medicare for their health needs. These men and women are not going to die soon. In fact, by 2025, these folks will make up 21 percent of the population and will be over seventy-five years old. Many are fit, healthy, and enjoying their retirement years well into their nineties — unlike healthcare, which is heading in the opposite direction. So, as healthy as you are, if you are part of this generation and are using or will be using this unhealthy healthcare system, you need to know how to protect yourself.

I met a 104-year-old patient. She was as spry and young as a seventy-year-old. I asked her what her secret was. She said that when she was in her fifties, she asked her doctor how to keep young and healthy. He told her there were three things she needed to do daily. Drink lots of water, get up and move every day to keep the body going, and surround herself with lots of friends.

She said she has lived by that advice. She has also found that taking each day as an adventure and waiting to see the excitement and friends she will meet as the day goes on has helped tremendously in her ability to stay young. She reminded me of my childhood, when we looked to each day with a sense of adventure and didn't worry about the rest.

CHAPTER 12

Why You Need a Certified Patient Advocate

Let's first agree that your health and healthcare don't retire. And who knows what healthcare is going to look like in ten, twenty, or thirty years from now? Already artificial intelligence (AI) has taken over some parts of medicine.

Hospitals are telling radiologists that computers can spot abnormal readings on x-rays, CT scans, and MRIs better than humans can, so they are asking radiologists to go by AI results and refrain from changing a diagnosis even though they may think differently based on personal knowledge the physician has about the patient.

Unfortunately, health cannot be saved up like money for a rainy day. Time marches on and so does your health. It is best to keep it finely tuned. If we keep swimming, we are going to tire. If we grab a float, we can take a breather. Are your floats in place?

Since you can't save up your health for the golden years, how will you use what you just learned in the first two parts of this book to get you through your later years? Easy; what you learned in this book are principles. The basics. They are not going away. They are founded on trust, transparency, communication, clarity, and concern for other human beings. Since the beginning of mankind, these principles have not changed.

You can make this time of life work for you if you are willing to keep your own records updated. Keep all your appointments, eat better, walk more, maintain a social life, and ask the right questions. Spend more time with family and find the things you always wanted to do "someday" but never got around to.

Let's go live our lives and not worry about healthcare. How do you do that? Well, it depends whether you're willing to spend the time necessary to navigate the system by yourself, or you want your son or daughter to do it for you, or you want to hire a professional care coordinator. The healthcare system is not going to change or go away. You will only stay frustrated if you think it will get better.

Consider this: Healthcare is a pressure cooker. It has thrown doctors and patients into the pot. And boy! Are we ever getting cooked! Think of patient advocates as the pressure-release valve.

You're going to need your doctors more and more as you age, so start looking at backups. Why would you need backups? Well, all of us have had our doctors quit our healthcare facility. In fact, one hospital lost seventy-plus providers in the first three months after announcing that doctors were getting their commissions cut. So bear in mind that your doctor, whom you like, may not be around very long.

And even if you had all the doctors in the world, what about your buddies? The baby boomers are the largest population of aging folks there has ever been. With 11,006 turning sixty-five each day until 2029, the population of America is aging quickly. Doctor's offices will be crammed, overbooked, and underpaid, with no time for breaks to restore resilience. As previously stated, by 2050, 21 percent of the American population will be over seventy-five and going strong! The average age in my urgent care was eighty-six.

If AI is going to determine your diagnosis, then your treatment plan is not far from being determined by AI as well. So, will you get the best diagnosis and the best treatment plan? In theory, yes. In reality, no! Why? Let's look at two reasons:

1) What drives healthcare today? Good practice or money? Common sense dictates that the programmers who will write AI will also be influ-

enced by the companies who make products for your treatment plans. So if AI indicates you have a broken hip, what is to stop it from suggesting an MRI from XYZ Company versus an x-ray, which would keep the cost down?

2) Doctors know that every patient is different and responds to treatment differently. No one knows their body better than the patient. So, how can AI, which crunches numbers and statistics all day long, tell you what is right for you? Are you average? Most patients are not. They are humans and have a right to be treated with what works best for them.

The next thought should be, how am I going to fight this? You can, and the good news is, you have three options:

Plan A. That's right — get yourself set up with your own medical records and get prepared for those emergencies. Understand that AI is coming and coming fast.

In Plan A you must evaluate your health and your options every six months. What's changing in your health? What needs to be better and what can't you change?

How about that insurance? Review and/or change your policy at least once a year. Are you going to the right pharmacy? Are you seeking the right doctors? Are you liking your doctors or just not bothering to change because it's too much trouble?

Let's say you decide to do this yourself. Set a schedule in six months to have this pop up on your phone with a date to get your self-review completed.

Let's say you did, but then you forgot about it. Let's go to Plan B.

Plan B. Call you daughter and have her review your medical chart, insurance, and make sure you have doctors and records all prepared with a backup plan.

Oh, but wait, you don't want to bother your daughter? Not a problem, let's go to Plan C.

Plan C. Hire a care coordinator to do this for you. Better yet, why not have someone you keep on a recurring monthly basis to review your records and keep them updated for you? "Oh, would you?" you say to that care coordinator. "Sure! This is what I do!"

Note that patient advocates do not call the people they work for patients, but clients. The reason stems from the fact that patient advocates are not hired to give, nor should they give, medical advice. They are there to guide the person through a fragmented healthcare system. Nor are patient advocates practicing law. Should someone need the services of a lawyer, the patient advocate often knows who the best attorneys in the community are who specialize in what their client needs.

Sometimes a social worker or nurse is employed by the hospital or clinic or emergency department to guide the patient after care is complete. The problem is that this patient advocate or navigator may be overwhelmed with the workload. If this is the case, get yourself your own advocate and pay the person out of your own pocket. They are well worth it for your emotional well-being and health safety. None of us can think well when under stress, in pain, or worried. Let someone else carry you during this time. You will be so glad to have this expertise. They know how medical errors occur, leaving you injured. They build relationships with your doctor. They want you to build that same trust. Since they are paid by you, they have a fiduciary responsibility to protect you from harm. They will never cover up a mistake for the benefit of big-business healthcare. While hospital-hired advocates also have your best interest at heart, they do not know you the way your own private advocate does. They cannot give you the service you truly need. After you leave a hospital or facility, they are done with you.

CHAPTER 13

When Our Children Become Our Parents

Many years ago, it was a fact of life that people really didn't live very long. I mean they retired at fifty-five or sixty-five and carried on for about eighteen months. Over the years, medicine changed, and soon we were looking at *On Golden Pond*. Everyone could live a long, healthy life and have a cabin to hide out in. The average age of patients in many medical practices today in Florida is over eighty.

Geriatric medicine emerged, and patients started seeking out gerontologists to tell them about dementia, disability, and death. If you expect to live very long, it would really behoove you to put the right doctors in place.

Every year I see the worst of the worst happen. A son or daughter decides that Mom or Dad can't take care of her- or himself anymore. So they tell the surviving parent to sell his or her home and return north to the cold, gray weather and freezing rain to live for all twelve months of the year. The aging parent must leave his home, his friends, his golfing buddies, his social amenities and all the personal and private activities his children knew nothing about. His daughters will fix a room for Pops in the house and he can live there. Maybe Pops doesn't want to go. Maybe Pops is just fine living at home in another part of the country. Why move?

It gets even worse. One aging parent and his wife told me that living away from their kids meant hanging out with friends they have known for years: "It's college without the exams." Well, some of us remember that experience and it got wild!

How do you get a feuding parent and adult child to act like grownups? When did the child become the parent? Who gave the child permission? The adult child is fraught with fear and emotion about losing her parent. The parent is feeling guilty about asking the adult child for help.

Here's how this happens. The son or daughter grows up, gets married or finds a life partner, gets a career, and may even has a few kids. The kids head off to school. The adult children are still working but call weekly to talk to their parents. Now the parents notice that instead of things like, "Mom, we are going to have another baby," or "Dad, I'm getting married," or "Dad, I'm switching jobs," or "Mom, I met someone," the conversation slowly turns to "Mom, what's that mark on your leg?" "Dad, why are the dishes in the sink?" "Dad, what did you eat today?" "Mom, we need to see the doctor because you are falling."

Here's Mom: "No, I am not falling and leave me alone." Here's Dad: "Look, I was putting up the rafters when I fell." And the response may be "Dad, you are too old to be on a ladder," . . . and so it goes. The child becomes the parent and the enjoyment of phoning the kids becomes onerous.

One of the major things I teach care coordinators, patient advocates, and adult children and friends of seniors is to remember to respect our aging population, the patient, regarding all decisions and plans.

When my daughter was turning sixteen, I tried teaching her how to read a map. How anyone could drive a car and not read a map was beyond my comprehension. Finally, I gave up and bought her the GPS system she kept talking about. She soon had her license and GPS, and off she went in her grandmother's old Buick. Six months passed and one day I asked her how she liked her GPS contraption. She said she *loved* it. Not really understanding how it worked, I asked her what she liked about it. She looked at me sheepishly and said, "You know, Mom, when I miss my turn or I go left instead of right, it doesn't yell at me; it doesn't make grunting noises. All it says is, 'Recalculating!'"

At that moment the lightbulb went on! When we work with others, shouldn't we just "recalculate"? As I have worked with hundreds of students, patients, and clients over the years, I just recalculate, and I ask their adult children or caretakers to just recalculate. It's no big deal if Mom doesn't want to go to the planned picnic when you arrive to take her. Just recalculate for another day. Find a new route, a new day, a new time. It's not a big deal. We all have days when we lack energy.

Enter the professional care coordinator who can understand this principle and see and amend both sides of this paradox. First, the care coordinator can assess the situation and see if Pops is really safe and functional in his own home. The advocate can also keep the family involved and informed. No surprises here. If Pops is not feeling well, then the care coordinator can discuss the next steps and the services that are needed.

Next, the care coordinator helps the aging parent decide what kind and extent of care and services he or she can afford.

The caregiver oversees all the special services, so someone "has eyes on" Pops. Let's say Pops goes to the doctor; the care coordinator can go too and let the doctor know much more about the patient and his safe living arrangements. Also, the professional patient advocate can let the family know what the doctor says. This is an easy enough agreement. Pops gets to stay in his home and community while the kids get regular updates about what is happening.

Let's look at another situation. Mom and Dad are doing just fine, but they feel their house is too much to care for anymore and want maintenance-free living. They look around the area and decide on a fancy, resort-type retirement community where they can afford to live. Mom and Dad go for a site visit. They are served the best filet mignon in the place. The place shows them all the bells and whistles.

Then comes the hard sell. "You'd better get in now or you won't have a place later. We only take healthy people and if you get sick later we can't guarantee you a spot." Mom is afraid she won't get into the joint, so she tells Dad they have to move. Dad likes their home and wants to stay and be able to fidget in the garden, trim the lawn, and give the neighbors a onceover. Nope, Mom will have none of it, and the next thing they know the house in on the market and they are moving. When were they going to tell the kids?

Now they have arrived in their new home. Depression sets in. Where are the filet mignon and all the trimmings, trappings, and social activities? Oh, sorry. The place has just changed hands; it's been bought out by a larger business, and those things are being eliminated. Wait, we must get out of this disaster. Nope. You sold your home. You are stuck. This happens all the time.

There are professional patient advocates out there who specialize in scouring the earth to find the right places to live after retirement and make sure those places are not being sold to big business. Their services are free of charge and they do incredible work to find you a nice place to live when you are ready to move, not a day before. There are no pressure tactics. How do we know the good guys from the bad? Easy, that's what patient coordinators do within their community. They find the best services for their clients; they are honest, trustworthy people.

Now let's not get started on "Honest people are hard to find." If we go down that road, there's nothing there for any of us. In fact, it's a dead end and we are all trapped. Life is changing. People are not as honest as they appear, and the handshake as a guarantee disappeared when the attorney showed up to do the contract. Adversarial conflict arose so certain professions could keep their mediation jobs. The news media loves a scandal. Social media loves it, too.

CHAPTER 14

The New Medical Practices Emerging for Better Healthcare

L et's be clear in our definitions.

Direct primary care (DPC) and concierge medicine are rapidly growing models of primary care found within family practice. Though the terms are used interchangeably, they are not the same. Such liberal use of terms, even within the industry, confuses those who are attempting to understand how these primary care models operate. It is not the fees that define these terms, but the way these physicians accept payment. I have attempted to differentiate between the two and then throw in a hybrid version.

> One doctor was fired from her practice because she would not see more patients. She felt she was not giving the best care. She eventually opened her own practice as a direct primary care physician.

Direct Primary Care

This is the fastest-growing type of medical practice today. With the direct primary care model, providers do not take insurance at all, but rather rely solely on a monthly or annual fee from patients.

The big benefit here for both you and your doctor is that the doctor is able to keep her or his practice small and tailored to the number of patients the doctor wishes to see.

As far as pros and cons, they are fairly reversed from the concierge model, which we will discuss next. A key benefit from not taking insurance is that the practice is not subject to many regulations. The practice also does not have to concern itself with contracting and credentialing with insurance companies, nor worry over denials, precertification, collecting co-pays, and so on. The doctor can also call the shots and keep the practice small. One direct primary care physician said he only needed forty-five patients paying $100 a month for him to cover his costs. Patients over that number provided his income. He preferred to keep his practice to one hundred families.

Unlike insurance-driven practices, these practices have no additional mandates. Providers have to be licensed to practice in their respective states, as in the 1950s to 1970s. However, they do not need to satisfy the 178 insurance mandates. This keeps their overhead low and they pass this saving on to their patients. They do not have billers, coders, nurses, and charting requirements. Time is spent seeing their patients for forty-five to sixty minutes on each visit. They love taking care of the patient and practicing medicine. They do not have to send out surveys to ask about customer satisfaction, because they know their patients love working with them.

The patient has access to the physician any time and often knows the staff personally. The physician is on call 24/7 for you. The physician may also provide labs and medications at a fraction of the cost of traditional healthcare. Not filing insurance, the doctor is not influenced to work under commission. The patient needs insurance only for hospitalizations, specialists, or emergency room visits, but the goal of your direct primary care doctor is to keep you healthy and out of emergency rooms and hospitals. This doctor can treat you for all sorts of disorders and diseases. You do not have to be sent to a "specialist," as the goal here is that this doctor-patient relationship remain intact and stable. Should you need a specialist, the direct primary care physician can call one and get the help needed, just like in the old days. Transparency and clarity drive this relationship.

Know that this provider typically needs thirty-five to four hundred patients to pay in each month to stay in business. Compare this to the two thousand patients healthcare requires their employed doctors to have. Liability insurance, continuing medical education, and medical board licensing are the three most expensive costs the provider must incur.

If you have a direct primary care physician, then I strongly recommend you keep that relationship, as these practices are filling up rather quickly.

According to figures currently available at the *Journal of American Boards of Family Medicine* online, for direct primary care you are looking at a median monthly cost of $75, with a range from about $27 to about $563. Practices that used the phrase "direct primary care" on average charged a lower fee than practices that used the term "*concierge*" to describe their model: about $77 compared with about $183, respectively. Of 116 practices with available price information, 28 (24 percent) charged a per-visit fee, and the average per-visit charge among this group was $15.59 (range, $5 to $35). Thirty-six of these 116 practices charged a one-time initial enrollment fee, and the average enrollment fee among this group was about $78 (range, $29 to $300).[1]

A drawback for these practices, however, is that there is only one source of revenue: the patient. Consequently, the practice must be diligent with its financial planning to ensure that patient fees are enough to support the practice operations.

Concierge Care

There are many varieties of concierge medicine, but in the traditional form the patient pays a monthly or annual fee for direct access to the physician. The practice not only profits from this fee but *also bills insurance companies for visits. This is the difference between direct primary care and concierge care.*[2]

On the financial side, these practices may collect money from two streams of revenue and thus not be as concerned with fighting insurance companies (for their only source of revenue) as they would in a traditional healthcare medical practice.

Typically, concierge medicine charges a higher monthly fee higher than the direct primary care provider. Their fees can start at $300 to $30,000 a month. While you will get the privilege of seeing your doctor within one to two days of calling, you will still spend only ten to fifteen minutes with your provider.

One key drawback of the concierge model is that if the provider is still accepting Medicare (or commercial payers with nondiscrimination clauses in their contracts), then the provider is subject to those government regulations for payment and the other 178 mandates of federal law. This paperwork and added charting leads to hiring scribes, billers, coders, and other personnel to keep the doors open. In some concierge offices, I saw that the $30,000-a-month patient gets to go through the back door to wait for the doctor. The exam room is built with crown molding and furnished with couches and lounge chairs for the patient.

The second drawback is that this physician may be working for large healthcare facilities that dictate how many patients the doctor can take, which can once again be overwhelming for the doctor. Patient panels can be as high as 1,500 patients per doctor. There may or may not be physician cell phone access or house call service.

For you, the patient, there are multiple questions you need to ask your doctor before signing up for concierge service. If you can afford the monthly fee, is there a signup fee, and is there an annual renewal fee above the monthly fee? Find out whether you will be directed to a call center or will have your call or text or email answered directly by your doctor.

Other questions deal with insurance: Will you have to file your own insurance papers? Who gets reimbursed? Will you need to carry catastrophic insurance over and above the monthly fee? What about labs, imaging studies, and extra orders given to you? Who pays for them and how much are they?

Last but not least, how is this provider paid? By the provider's employer, directly by monthly fees obtained through patients, or on commission? Does the doctor charge additional fees for services performed or medications provided in the office? For example, if lab orders require blood to be drawn and sent to the lab, are fees added to draw the blood on top of the lab fee? Can you, the patient, write off the monthly fees as a health expense? Your providers may not know this answer, so it is best to ask your tax advisor in the state where your concierge or direct primary care provider offers services.

Hybrid

The last model is a hybrid of a traditional practice and the concierge model. Essentially, providers with a hybrid model have a number of patients in the practice under the traditional model and a smaller set of patients that are under the concierge model. They are trying to convert over to a direct care model but cannot leave their revenue at this time.

A practical reason to go with this approach is that it allows the doctor to determine whether eventually going entirely off a traditional practice model is a viable option. Physicians also like this model because they are able to retain many of their established patients (under the insurance-payment side) without having to hand them off to another practice.

A key downside, however, is that this model takes a lot of operational planning and scheduling finesse because, simply put, patients paying a fee for concierge medicine expect to be at the front of the line. This means that if you are paying a monthly fee, you will get in to see the doctor in one or two days and bump someone else in the waiting room. This does not mean you do not have to wait. While your appointment may be at 3 p.m., your doctor may not see you until 5 p.m.

Another downside is that the practice still has a significant number of traditional patients, and thus it is subject to some of the insurance rules and regulations mentioned earlier, as well as the continued headaches of billing and collection. This is one of the reasons the doctor usually charges you a significant monthly fee; these doctors have to meet their overhead.

Confusion arises from similarities that exist between models, such as decreased patient panels, monthly subscriptions, and longer visits. There is added confusion when a DPC physician offers house calls or email access, typical of concierge practices. Confusion is maximized when a physician is by definition practicing direct primary care yet calls the practice a "concierge practice." Similarly, a concierge practice may decide to abstain from participating in third-party payer systems and thus would also be a DPC practice.

In summary, not all direct primary care practices are concierge practices, and not all concierge practices are direct primary care practices. The terms are not synonymous, and even the fundamentals of the two models do not overlap. The key to differentiation is whether or not a third-party payer is involved.

Decide whether traditional medicine or one of these above medical models is best for you.

Think about living each day to the fullest and surround yourself with the right people to help you continue to grow, laugh, and love. After all, you deserve it.

But we never know what life will throw at us. When life events do throw curves to our health or our aging, they put new pressure on us and our loved ones. Our energy — emotionally, physically, and mentally — will wax and wane. We at Patient Best®, LLC, want to stabilize our clients' lives. I am grateful to all the patient advocates who get up every day to help those who struggle with the unknowns, the expected, and the emergencies. I appreciate their hard work to pave the road for another family, to befriend a client and their family, and walk through life's hardest toll.

Healthcare does not have to be complicated. It should lift the burden of heartbreak, not contribute to it. Patient Best® advocates can be found at www.PatientBest.com. They personalize a service that helps you get the healthcare you deserve in the time you need it, with outcomes you understand and the clarity you hope for. They will guide you through those challenging, changing times.

Take Care. Stay Safe. Talk Soon.

Acknowledgments

I want to thank all the wonderful patients, physicians, nurses, nurse practitioners, and physician assistants who have helped me become a better practitioner and certified patient advocate. You took your valuable time to teach another and I have learned so much. My hope is that I can pass your wisdom on to those who come behind me.

Special thanks to the following Patient Best® advocates who have brought so much of this book into fruition with their dedication, skill, knowledge, time, stories, and solutions:

Kathleen McMillan, PharmD, of Ft Myers Beach, FL, who has helped many patients stay safe in the healthcare system. Your wealth of knowledge and understanding of the medical charts, rules, and regulations has brought so much peace of mind to your clients and their families. So many wrong turns have been prevented under your guidance. Thank you for sharing and caring.

Sue Roseliep, of Naples, FL, who specializes in long-term insurance and transitioning patients to safe and more appropriate living places. You have brought such peace to so many families. Your perfect timing and wisdom make you a hero for so many loved ones. Your skill in discerning services for those you care for exemplifies the love you have for your profession and your clients.

Pamela Edmonds, of Hartford, CT, who specializes in health insurance and medical billing. You have saved thousands of dollars and headaches for your clients. Your commitment to seek out and find a solution to the mountain of paperwork, unanswered phone calls, and misdirected explanations has led to recovering thousands of dollars for your clients. No one should have to suffer this kind of financial loss. You are there to oversee these bills every step of the way and customize their health insurance to fit their needs.

And thanks to my copy editor, Martha Woolverton, who spent countless hours reading and rereading this material with patience and care so the final product would come together flawlessly.

Special thanks to my designer, Christy Collins, who took her skill, knowledge, and time to bring her best and creative ideas forthwith to introduce this book to you all.

May safe health be the norm in our futures!

Notes

Chapter 2

1. With the da Vinci Surgical System, surgeons operate through just a few small incisions. The da Vinci System features a magnified 3-D high-definition vision system and tiny wristed instruments that bend and rotate to a far greater extent than the human hand. As a result, da Vinci enables your surgeon to operate with enhanced vision, precision, and control. See "Da Vinci® Surgery: Minimally Invasive Surgery." Da Vinci Surgery — Minimally Invasive Robotic Surgery with the Da Vinci Surgical System. Accessed November 14, 2018. http://www.davincisurgery.com/.

2. Jerome E. Groopman, *How Doctors Think*. Boston: Houghton Mifflin, 2011.

3. National Patient Safety Foundation, "Preventable Health Care Harm Is a Public Crisis." Role of the Patient Advocate — Institute for Healthcare Improvement. March 13, 2013. Accessed November 14, 2018. https://www.npsf.org/page/public_health_crisis.

4. Vanessa McMains, "Johns Hopkins Study Suggests Medical Errors Are Third-leading Cause of Death in U.S." The Hub. May 03, 2016. Accessed November 14, 2018. https://hub.jhu.edu/2016/05/03/medical-errors-third-leading-cause-of-death/.

Chapter 3

1. Groopman, *How Doctors Think* (see ch. 2, note 2).

2. Jim Loehr and Tony Schwartz, *The Power of Full Engagement: Managing Energy, Not Time, Is the Key to High Performance and Personal Renewal.* Riverside: Free Press, 2005.

3. WWWebTek, Inc., The Harold P. Freeman Patient Navigation Institute. Accessed November 14, 2018. http://www.hpfreemanpni.org/.

4. Nicole Spector, "The Doctor Is Out? Why Physicians Are Leaving Their Practices to Pursue Other Careers." NBCNews.com. Accessed November 14, 2018. https://www.nbcnews.com/business/business-news/doctor-out-why-physicians-are-leaving-their-practices-pursue-other-n900921.

5. Chad Terhune, "Americans Waste $200 Billion Every Year on Medical Tests They Don't Need, Experts Say." Los Angeles Times. May 25, 2017. Accessed November 14, 2018. http://www.latimes.com/business/la-fi-medical-tests-20170526-story.html.

6. "What Is Care Coordination?" NEJM Catalyst. September 25, 2018. Accessed November 14, 2018. https://catalyst.nejm.org/what-is-care-coordination/.

Chapter 5

1. In a research study conducted by physician assistant students at the University of Kentucky, over 70% of one emergency room's charts had wrong telephone numbers, leaving staff frustrated that they could not contact patients with follow-up instructions or appointments.
Personal communication. Per this website: https://libguides.murdoch.edu.au/Chicago/personal.

Chapter 6

1. Milton Packer, "How to Stop Direct-to-Consumer Prescription Drug Ads." Medpage Today. May 23, 2018. Accessed November 14, 2018. https://www.medpagetoday.com/blogs/revolutionandrevelation/73060.

2. Gina Chon, "Rising Drug Prices Put Big Pharma's Lobbying to the Test." New York Times. December 21, 2017. Accessed November 14, 2018. https://www.nytimes.com/2016/09/02/business/dealbook/rising-drug-prices-put-big-pharmas-lobbying-to-the-test.html.

Chapter 8

1. "Drugs Linked to Erectile Dysfunction." WebMD. Accessed November 14, 2018. https://www.webmd.com/erectile-dysfunction/guide/drugs-linked-erectile-dysfunction.

2. R. Weinick, J. Billings, and J. Thorpe, "Ambulatory Care Sensitive Emergency Department Visits: A National Perspective." Abstr AcademyHealth Meet, 2003:20, abstract no. 8. https://www.nehi.net/writable/publication_files/file/nehi_ed_overuse_issue_brief_032610finaledits.pdf.

3. "How Much Does an Emergency Room Visit Cost?" CostHelper. Accessed November 27, 2018. https://health.costhelper.com/emergency-room.html.

4. "Hearing Loss and Dementia — Who's Listening?" *Aging & Mental Health*. August 18, 2014.
https://www.tandfonline.com/doi/abs/10.1080/13607863.2014.915924?journalCode=camh20

5. "Lost Mothers: Maternal Mortality in the U.S." NPR. May 12, 2017. Accessed November 14, 2018. https://www.npr.org/series/543928389/lost-mothers.

6. Kimberly Amadeo, "See for Yourself If Obamacare Increased Health Care Costs." The Balance Small Business. Accessed November 14, 2018. https://www.thebalance.com/causes-of-rising-healthcare-costs-4064878.

Chapter 14

1. Philip M. Eskew, "Philip M. Eskew." *Journal of the American Board of Family Medicine*. June 14, 2015. Accessed November 14, 2018. http://www.jabfm.org/content/28/6/793.

2. Nick Hernandez, "Concierge Medicine vs Direct Primary Care." January 28, 2015. Accessed November 14, 2018. http://www.bibme.org/chicago/website-citation/search?utf8=&q=http://www.physicianspractice.com/fee-schedule-survey/concierge-medicine-vs-direct-primary-care.

www.ingramcontent.com/pod-product-compliance
Lightning Source LLC
Chambersburg PA
CBHW021336290326
41933CB00038B/776